GW01255632

For Elsevier:

Associate Editor: Siobhan Campbell
Development: Veronika Krcilova
Project Manager: Gail Wright
Senior Designer: George Ajayi
Illustration Manager: Bruce Hogarth

Practical Electrotherapy
A guide to safe application

John Fox MSc MCSP
Lecturer, Department of Physiotherapy,
University of Cardiff, Cardiff, UK

Tim Sharp BSc(Hons) MCSP
Lecturer, Department of Physiotherapy,
University of Cardiff, Cardiff, UK

FOREWORD BY

Sheila Kitchen PhD MSc MSCP DipTp
Head of Department,
Academic Department of Physiotherapy,
School of Biomedical and Health Sciences,
Guy's Campus,
London, UK

CHURCHILL LIVINGSTONE

ELSEVIER

Edinburgh London New York Oxford Philadelphia
St Louis Sydney Toronto 2007

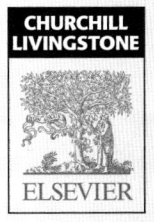

CHURCHILL
LIVINGSTONE
ELSEVIER

First published 2007

© 2007, Elsevier Limited. All rights reserved.

No part of this publication may be reproduced, stored in a retrieval system, or transmitted in any form or by any means, electronic, mechanical, photocopying, recording or otherwise, without the prior permission of the Publishers. Permissions may be sought directly from Elsevier's Health Sciences Rights Department, 1600 John F. Kennedy Boulevard, Suite 1800, Philadelphia, PA 19103-2899, USA: phone: (+1) 215 239 3804; fax: (+1) 215 239 3805; or, e-mail: healthpermissions@elsevier.com. You may also complete your request on-line via the Elsevier homepage (http://www.elsevier.com), by selecting 'Support and contact' and then 'Copyright and Permission'.

ISBN: 978-0-443-06855-3

British Library Cataloguing in Publication Data
A catalogue record for this book is available from the British Library

Library of Congress Cataloging in Publication Data
A catalog record for this book is available from the Library of Congress

Note
Neither the Publisher nor the Authors assume any responsibility for any loss or injury and/or damage to persons or property arising out of or related to any use of the material contained in this book. It is the responsibility of the treating practitioner, relying on independent expertise and knowledge of the patient, to determine the best treatment and method of application for the patient.

The Publisher

Working together to grow
libraries in developing countries

www.elsevier.com | www.bookaid.org | www.sabre.org

ELSEVIER   BOOK AID International   Sabre Foundation

your source for books,
journals and multimedia
in the health sciences

www.elsevierhealth.com

The publisher's policy is to use paper manufactured from sustainable forests

Printed in China

Contents

Foreword vii

Preface xi

Acknowledgements xv

PART 1 – HEATING AND COOLING   1

Chapter 1   Hydrocollator (hot) packs   3
Chapter 2   Paraffin wax bath   17
Chapter 3   Shortwave diathermy   31
Chapter 4   Ice/cold packs (cryotherapy)   53

PART 2 – ELECTRICAL STIMULATION   75

Chapter 5   Transcutaneous electrical nerve stimulation   77
Chapter 6   Neuromuscular electrical stimulation   103
Chapter 7   Interferential therapy   137

PART 3 – BIOSTIMULATION OF TISSUE   157

Chapter 8   Pulsed shortwave diathermy   159
Chapter 9   Ultrasound therapy   185
Chapter 10 Laser therapy   213

Appendix 1: Electrical safety   237

Appendix 2: Electrotherapeutic parameters   241

Appendix 3: Electrotherapy: skin sensation testing   243

Index   245

Foreword

INTRODUCTION

This book has been developed by John Fox and Tim Sharp to provide a very useful and practical guide to the use of electrotherapeutic agents – and will be particularly valuable to students who are practicing their techniques or who find themselves in a practice setting and needing help with the selection and application of a treatment. It is detailed, clear and covers most techniques that students from a variety of backgrounds may need in their practice.

'Electrotherapy' is a generic term covering a wide variety of therapies – not all of which are actually 'electrically' based (e.g. many forms of cooling) or therapeutic (some are primarily used for testing or monitoring). The term covers modalities that physiotherapists and others have used as part of their repertoire since the earliest days of their practice as well as more recent introductions. The use of some agents such as heat, cold and some forms of electrical stimulation have a reasonable, though still often limited, evidence base for their use, while others are less securely evidenced. This means that – in line with many treatments for a wide variety of conditions used by many professions – the student/practitioner cannot use a 'cook book' approach to selecting, using and evaluating these interventions. Such an approach is unlikely to lead to best, evidence-based practice that is effective, efficient and economical. In contrast, the reader must weigh up all the evidence (see below) to inform their selection and usage of electrophysical treatments, and be prepared to reflect on the outcome critically as they progress.

DESIGN AND STYLE OF BOOK

This book is designed primarily to provide the reader with key information to guide them when making decisions about the safe and effective use of electrophysical treatments. The authors of this book describe a safe process for the application of the most common treatments that are in current use, provide basic physical and physiological information about possible effects and hazards, and provide summaries of a number of research studies that have investigated the efficacy of the treatments in a variety of situations. Instructions for application are detailed. In addition, they provide the reader with a checklist that can be used to trigger reflection on the effects of the intervention with a view to informing future care.

HOW TO USE THIS BOOK

However, this book cannot be used to support best practice without considerable 'work' on the part of the reader – work that is a normal and necessary part of clinical practice. This is not a cook book. It is essential that the information presented so very clearly is used as part of the clinical reasoning process as the reader selects the appropriate treatment modality, the dosage and then evaluates and progresses the treatment.

The key, interconnected concepts underpinning all clinical practice are presented in Figure 1, and involve the use of evidence to inform decision making through clinical reasoning.

The student/practitioner needs full information about the client/patient, including factors such as:

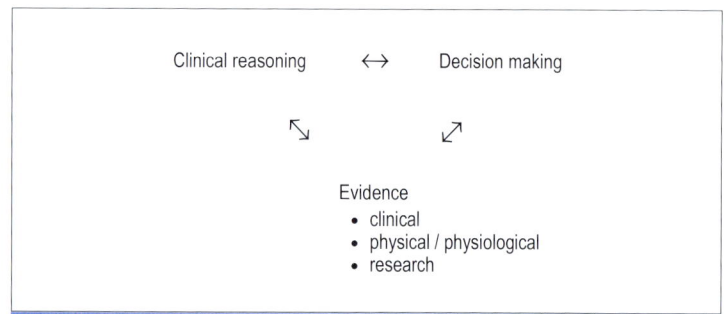

Figure 1 The relationship between evidence, clinical reasoning and decision making.

- the needs (physical, functional, social and psychological) of the client/patient
- their diagnosis and symptoms
- the underlying pathology of the presenting condition and repair processes
- the course of the condition; for example, acute, chronic, resolving, fluctuating, etc.
- factors exacerbating or relieving the condition or symptoms.

With this information a reasoned decision can be made about the therapeutic effects that are desirable. Information is then needed about the therapeutic agents that might be used, including:

- the physical effects known to result from the treatment under consideration; for example, will it penetrate deeply enough to reach the target tissue?
- the physiological effects of the treatment being considered; does it slow down repair (e.g. cold), speed up processes (e.g. heat) or stimulate nerve conduction?
- the evidence for the efficacy of this treatment for the condition in question, or for similar conditions. Is there any evidence that this treatment is beneficial – beyond the normal rates of repair or improvement? What dose is thought/known to be effective? How often should it be given?
- any hazards that are associated with its use, and safety precautions that should be considered.

The information gathered will in turn lead to a decision about the possible therapeutic effects that are likely to occur. This process is summarised below (Fig. 2) in a model of clinical decision making in electrotherapy, adapted from Watson (2000).

CLINICAL DECISION MAKING

⇕

Theory   Physical effects ↔ Physiological effects ↔ Therapeutic effects   Client

⇕

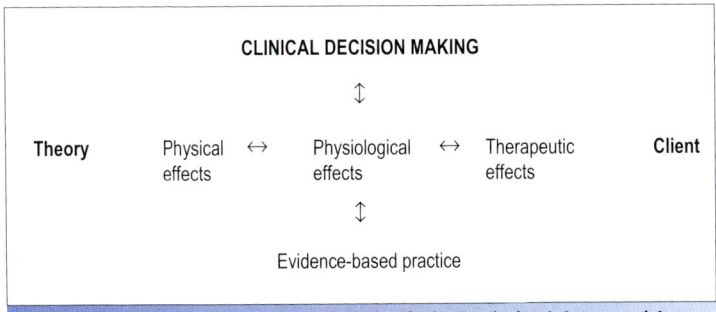

Evidence-based practice

Figure 2 An integrated model of clinical decision making in electrotherapy.

Evidence of efficacy is a constantly shifting body of knowledge, and is gathered from a wide variety of sources:

- Clinical information: past experience with other patients, talking and listening to them and reflection on their responses – physical/physiological, and functional – provide useful guidance.
- Basic physical and physiological information: what does the basic scientific knowledge suggest that the benefits of this treatment should/might be?
- Research evidence: clinical and laboratory studies, reviews (such as those undertaken by Cochrane review teams) and audit reports are all used to inform practice.

All of this information needs to be critically reviewed and integrated to inform your clinical decision about the treatment to be used. This book provides the reader with a snapshot of a number of research papers currently available addressing the use of each agent described. It provides key points to remind the reader of the factors they need to consider in terms of the basic physical and physiological principles but obviously cannot provide information derived from clinical experience. However, the key probes to help in your reflection about interventions will be very useful in helping to build up this aspect.

It is essential that the reader updates this material regularly for themselves, reviews the quality of the research papers presented here and any material identified and draws reasoned conclusions before selecting a treatment. This information then needs to be integrated in the process we call clinical reasoning to make an informed judgement about the best options for a given person and condition.

CONCLUSION

This book provides you with key points to direct your reasoning, detailed and safe guidelines for administering the treatment and probes to stimulate reflection on your intervention. It does not – and should not! – absolve you from the responsibility of making informed decisions. This responsibility is yours!

REFERENCE

Watson T 2000 The role of electrotherapy in contemporary physiotherapy practice. Manual Therapy 5(3):132–141

Preface

The foundations of this book arose from teaching electrotherapy to undergraduate physiotherapy students. Despite the numerous scientific texts around, none of them informed the students of what they needed to know when faced with a machine which they had seen and used in the past, but could not quite remember what all the buttons were for. As a supplement to the teaching these individual guides were borne which proved popular and useful. The next logical step was to collate the various parts and make them into a book. Fortunately for us, the need for such a publication appeared much greater than we had anticipated.

From the outset this book was designed to be a practical guide. It is not intended to be used for clinical decision making regarding best practice. We recommend that this book is supplemented with a standard electrotherapy text such as *Electrotherapy explained* by Robertson et al (2006) or *Electrotherapy: evidence-based practice* edited by Sheila Kitchen (2002). The Chartered Society of Physiotherapy (CSP) has just recently issued a publication entitled 'Guidance for the clinical use of electrotherapy agents' (2006). However, that is not to say that this book lacks any theoretical principles or physiological rationale. To allow safe application some knowledge of the physiological effects and the possible dangers and contraindications is essential. Some information on these aspects has been included.

To supplement the teaching within the classroom we found that peer observation was very effective at enhancing understanding. The peer observation checklist helps to structure the observation but is equally effective as an aid to reflection. Alongside this is space in which to record a simulated patient record and an area to write down any notes on the finer intricacies of the application.

There are a multitude of different machines and it is impossible to represent all of the different manufacturers and machines. Where possible we have included some different types of machines.

THE PATIENT'S STATE OF READINESS

The patient is welcomed by the physiotherapist, who gives the patient their full name and escorts them to the treatment cubicle. The treatment cubicle, usually a curtained area, should have been tidied and prepared with a pillow, blanket, chair, etc. It may be appropriate in some circumstances to assess/treat your patient in a separate room. It is important to remember that if your patient has a pacemaker they are not allowed within three metres of an operating shortwave diathermy machine.

The patient is told the examination/assessment will take about 40 minutes. A thorough subjective and objective assessment should be performed. The patient should be appropriately clothed; making sure the area you are assessing/treating is suitably exposed. An area cannot be adequately examined or treated through clothing. It is very important to use a blanket to maintain the modesty of the patient. Any jewellery or a watch should be removed prior to assessment/treatment.

After the initial assessment a treatment plan is formulated and this is discussed with the patient. The patient is given a full explanation of the treatment that has been recommended. The patient must consent to this treatment plan before continuing. If an electrotherapy modality is going to be employed then we need to ascertain if the patient has any contraindications to the modality.

The patient is made comfortable in a chair (or on the plinth) and the part to be treated must be fully supported. We may need to perform a skin sensation test if a heat treatment is being given or a pin-prick test if an electrical stimulation treatment is being given. When performing electrical stimulation we may need to clean the area to reduce skin impedance.

The 'machine' is tested to ensure it is working correctly. The plug and cable should be examined for any potential faults. The patient is 'set up' with safety uppermost (see individual sections). Again, if a heat treatment is being given then the patient is warned against the treatment getting too hot and causing a possible burn. They must just feel a 'mild comfortable warmth'. If the temperature does get too hot they must let the therapist know so they can turn down the temperature. The therapist should stay close at hand at all times throughout the treatment.

After the treatment has been completed the machine is turned off and all dials turned to zero. The skin is inspected and with a heat treatment there is usually a mild erythema present, but not a strong reaction. The patient may be given specific advice on home treatment and exercises, etc.

The therapist must then record the treatment: treatment received and time given, position of patient, explanation of treatment given, skin test performed, warning given, contraindications questioned, machine used, dosage given, any adverse reactions to treatment, date and signature.

ADDITIONAL READING

We have taken the opportunity to search out relative papers summarising studies investigating the effectiveness of all the electrotherapeutic modalities. This reflects, to some extent, the considerable amount of research that has been undertaken using electrotherapy modalities. These papers have been put into a table format and include brief descriptions of the aims, methods, assessment procedures and results. This is not a critical appraisal of the literature and therefore does not give an indication of the research quality. Most of the references are from papers readily available from the university or hospital library.

Chartered Society of Physiotherapy 2006 Guidance for the clinical use of electrotherapy agents.

Kitchen S 2002 Electrotherapy: evidence-based practice. Churchill Livingstone, London

Robertson V, Ward A, Low J, Reed A 2006 Electrotherapy explained: principles and practice, 4th edn. Elsevier, Oxford

Acknowledgements

We wish to thank our colleagues, whose encouragement and support has been invaluable throughout the writing of this publication. We are also grateful to Matthew Townsend, Richard Day, Karen Jones, Philippa Coales and Richard Paul-Taylor for their assistance in being willing subjects for the illustrations. We also wish to thank Michelle Evans and Tim Rebeiro for their technical support.

Lastly, we wish to thank the staff at Elsevier who initially encouraged the project and have patiently dealt with all our queries and concerns.

Cardiff 2006 *John Fox and Tim Sharp*

PART 1

HEATING AND COOLING

Chapter 1 – Hydrocollator (hot) packs	3
Chapter 2 – Paraffin wax bath	17
Chapter 3 – Shortwave diathermy	31
Chapter 4 – Ice/cold packs (cryotherapy)	53

CHAPTER 1

Hydrocollator (hot) packs

PRODUCTION

Hydrocollator (hot) packs produce their physiological effects through conduction. These silicate gel packs are kept in a hydrocollator tank, which is maintained at a temperature of 75–80°C. These packs are placed inside towel covers and then again wrapped in towelling. The towel provides some insulation, preventing the skin exceeding 40–42°C (Kitchen 2002, Robertson et al 2006).

EQUIPMENT

Hydrocollator (hot) pack
Tongs
Towels/towelling wrap
Tray
Blanket
Hot and cold test tubes for skin sensation (thermal) testing.

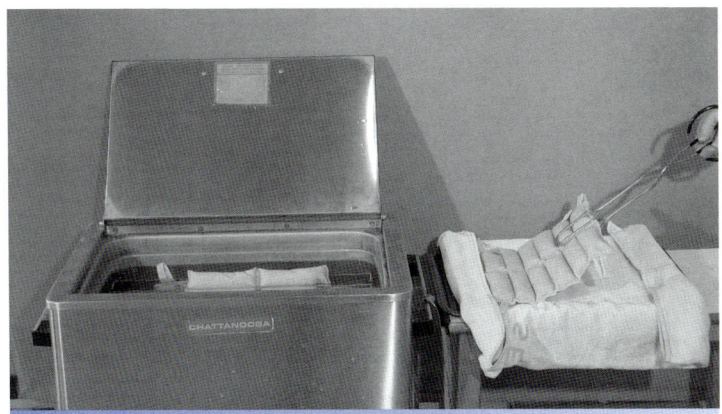

Figure 1.1 Hydrocollator and standard hot pack.

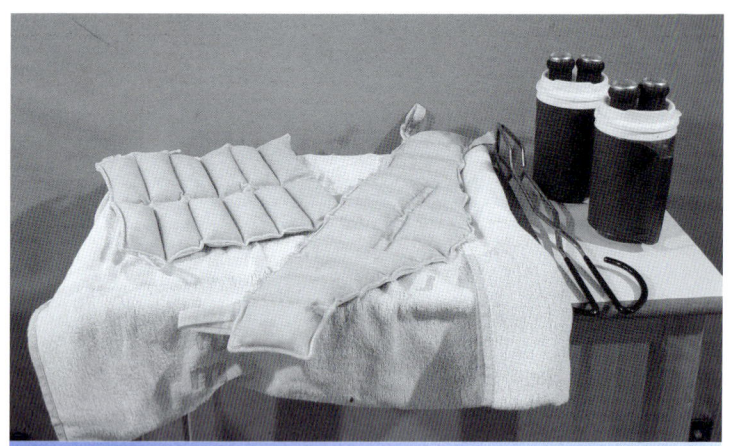

Figure 1.2 Hot packs, tongs, towels and hot and cold skin test kit.

APPLICATION TO THE LOW BACK

1. Remove upper garments. Position the patient prone on the plinth.
2. Beware if the patient has been using embrocation, e.g. deep heat, as this may cause a burn.
3. Explain the treatment and re-check for any contraindications.
4. Gain informed consent.
5. Perform a skin sensation (thermal) test over the area to be treated.
6. Remove pack from hydrocollator tank with tongs.
7. Wrap the hot pack in a towel (two layers) or Terry towelling cover.
8. Carry over to the patient on a tray.
9. If wrapping the hot pack with towels, add further layers to the hot pack so there are approximately eight layers, although this number will be dependent on the comfort of the patient.
10. Explain that it should be a mild, comfortable warmth and there is a possibility of a burn occurring if it is allowed to get too hot.
11. Apply the hot pack over the area to be treated.
12. Check the area after 5 min.
13. The temperature can be varied by varying the number of towelling layers between the patient and the hot pack.
14. After treatment, usually 15–20 min, check the area for any adverse reaction to treatment.

Hydrocollator (hot) packs

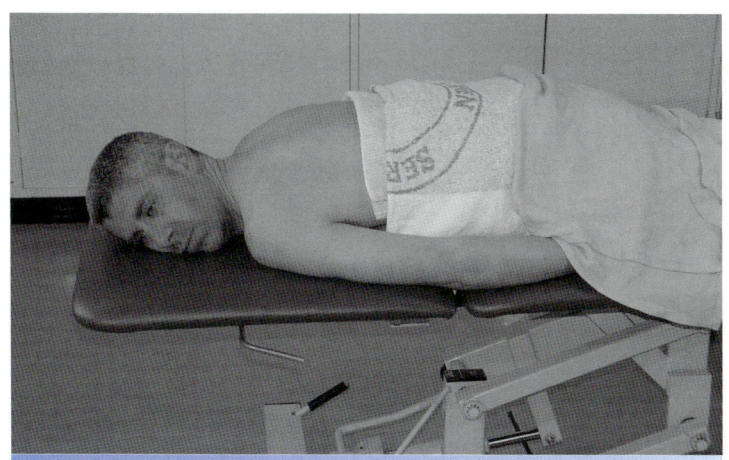

Figure 1.3 Hot pack to the lumbar spine. The hot pack is kept in position by placing a folded towel over the entire application and tucking it in under the patient.

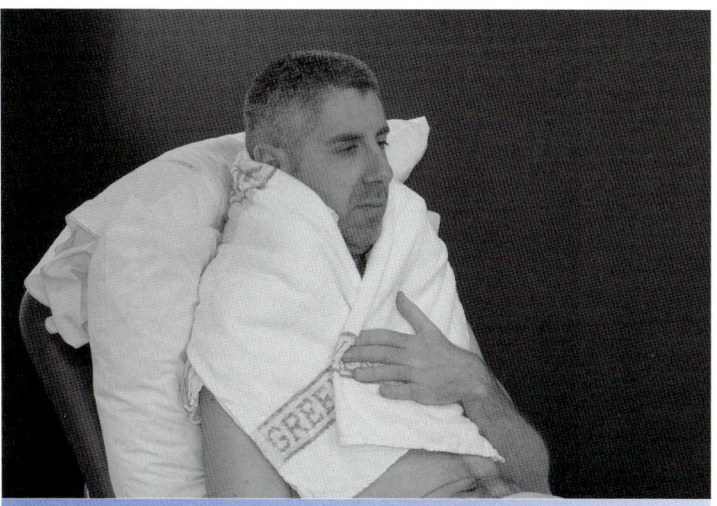

Figure 1.4 Illustration of hot pack to the cervical spine. The patient is fully supported in a half-lying position on the plinth. The hot pack is kept in place by positioning pillows to support the shoulders and head. The patient is not leaning with his full weight against the hot pack as this could cause a burn.

OTHER TYPES OF HOT PACKS

HEAT WRAP

Heat wrap is a lightweight, disposable, continuous low-level heating modality. The heat wrap is made of layers of cloth-like material that contain ingredients which produce heat on exposure to oxygen. The heat wrap reaches its therapeutic temperature of 40°C within 30 min and can deliver heat for up to 8 h (Mayer et al 2005). The heat wrap can be applied to the neck, low back and upper limbs. It allows heat application as the patient continues to be functionally active.

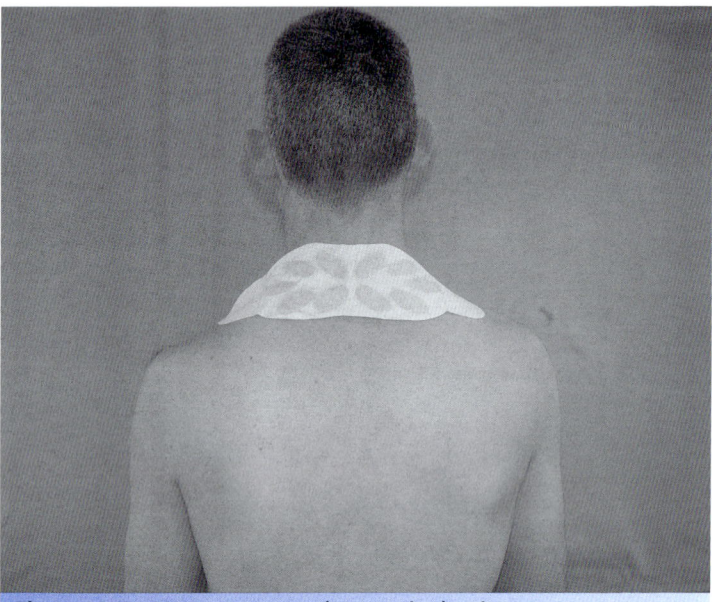

Figure 1.5 Heat wrap to the cervical spine.

Hydrocollator (hot) packs

Table 1.1 *PHYSIOLOGICAL EFFECTS, THERAPEUTIC USES AND CONTRAINDICATIONS AND PRECAUTIONS*

Physiological effects	Therapeutic uses	Contraindications/precautions
↑ Metabolic activity	Encourage healing ↑ Metabolic rate ↑ Phagocytosis ↑ Oxygen release and use	Infections Acute inflammation Skin tumours Acute skin disease
↑ Blood supply	↑ Nutrient and O_2 supply ↓ Metabolite ↓ Chemical pain mediators	Impaired blood supply Drowsy patient Deep X-ray therapy Local bleeding
↑ Tissue fluid exchange	↓ Oedema	Acute trauma
Nerve stimulation	Sensory/thermal: ↓ Pain Golgi tendon inhibition: ↓ Muscle spasm	
↓ Viscosity	↓ Peripheral resistance Synovial fluid: ↑ Joint range	Defective blood pressure regulation
↑ Extensibility of collagen	Precursor to stretching	

See also Robertson et al (2006).

Notes

Hydrocollator (hot) packs

Treatment record

Table 1.2 *OBSERVATIONAL/REFLECTIVE CHECKLIST*

	Observation	Y/N	Comments
Introduction	Did the therapist introduce him/herself?	☐	☐
	Was an explanation of the procedure given?	☐	☐
	Was the explanation clear and succinct?	☐	☐
	Were the possible dangers highlighted?	☐	☐
	Was consent obtained?	☐	☐
Comfort and safety	Was the patient comfortable?	☐	☐
	Was the therapist's posture compromised?	☐	☐
	Was the position safe for both parties?	☐	☐
	Was the modality applied with due care and attention?	☐	☐
Technique	Were the contraindications checked?	☐	☐
	Were the appropriate tests performed prior to treatment?	☐	☐
	Was an explanation of the physiological effects of the technique offered to the patient?	☐	☐
	Was this explanation accurate?	☐	☐
	Was the technique/modality applied correctly?	☐	☐
	Were the correct times and settings used?	☐	☐
	Was the skin checked after the treatment for adverse effects?	☐	☐

Hydrocollator (hot) packs

Table 1.3 *SUMMARY OF STUDIES INVESTIGATING THE EFFECTIVENESS OF HEAT TREATMENTS*

Authors	Aim of study	Numbers	Methods	Assessment	Results
Brosseau et al (2002)	The reviewers concluded that thermotherapy (hot packs, ice packs, paraffin wax baths and faradic baths) can be used as a palliative therapy, or as an adjunct therapy combined with exercise for rheumatoid arthritic patients; especially wax baths in the treatment of arthritic hands. They also said that the conclusions are limited by methodological considerations such as the poor quality of trials.				
French et al (2006)	To determine the efficacy of superficial heat or cold therapies in reducing pain and disability in low back pain in adults.	Nine trials involving 1117 participants were included in the review.	The authors undertook a systematic search of the literature. Nine studies were randomised controlled trials (RCTs) and were reviewed by the authors.		The authors concluded that there was moderate evidence that continuous heat wrap therapy reduced pain and disability in the short term. They said there was insufficient evidence about the effect of the application of cold for low back pain.
Kauranen & Vanharanta (1997)	To evaluate the effects of hot and cold packs on motor performance of normal hands.	20 healthy female students.	All subjects received a hot pack for 20 min to forearm and hand. They later received a cold pack for 15 min to the same area.	Four hand tests (reaction time, movement speed, tapping time and coordination), taken immediately, 15 min and 30 min after treatment.	Hot pack treatment delayed simple reaction time and increased tapping speed. Cold treatment delayed simple reaction time, speed of movement and tapping time.

Authors	Aim of study	Numbers	Methods	Assessment	Results
Mayer et al (2005)	To evaluate the efficacy of continuous low-level heat wrap therapy alone, combined with active exercises vs active exercises alone and control on the functional ability of patients with acute low back pain.	100 subjects with acute low back pain were randomised into four groups.	Group 1: (25 subjects) received heat wrap to wear for 8 h/day for 5 consecutive days. Group 2: (25 subjects) performed specific exercises, every hour during the day for 5 consecutive days. Group 3: (24 subjects) received heat wrap and exercises. Group 4: (26 subjects) were given a booklet on acute low back problems.	All participants were assessed by the Multidimensional Task Ability Profile Questionnaire and the Roland-Morris Disability Questionnaire.	The authors concluded that combining continuous low-level heat wrap therapy with directional preference-based exercises offered an advantage over either therapy alone for the treatment of acute low back pain.
Michlovitz et al (2004)	To determine the efficacy of continuous low-level heat wrap therapy compared with oral placebo treatment in subjects with wrist	93 patients with wrist pain (56 associated with SS, 13 with OA and 24 with CTS) were	Group 1: (39 subjects) received heat wrap to the wrist for 8 h. Group 2: (42 patients) received oral placebo. Group 3: (6 subjects) received active analgesia.	All participants were assessed for pain relief (0–5 verbal rating scale), joint stiffness (101-point numeric rating scale), grip strength and the Patient-	Heat wrap therapy showed significant benefits in day 1–3 mean pain relief ($p = 0.045$) and increased day 3 grip strength ($p = 0.02$) vs oral placebo for SS/T/OA groups. For the CTS group, heat wrap provided greater day 1–3 mean pain relief

Authors	Aim of study	Numbers	Methods	Assessment	Results
	pain due to strains and sprains (SS), tendinosis (T), osteoarthritis (OA), or carpal tunnel syndrome (CTS).	randomly assigned into four groups.	*Group 4:* (6 subjects) received an unheated heat wrap. Each participant had 3 consecutive days of treatment.	Rated Wrist Evaluation (PRWE). Patients with CTS also completed a symptom severity scale (SSS) and a functional status scale (FSS).	($p = 0.001$), day 1–3 mean joint stiffness reduction ($p = 0.004$), increased day 3 grip strength ($p = 0.003$), reduced PRWE scores and improved functional status ($p = 0.04$).
Nadler et al (2002)	To compare the efficacy of heat wrap to the maximum dosages of ibuprofen and acetaminophen for self-treatment of acute non-specific low back pain.	371 patients with acute non-specific low back pain were randomised into five groups.	*Group 1:* (113 subjects) received heat wrap to lumbar spine for 8 h. *Group 2:* (113 subjects) received oral acetaminophen (2 tablets, 4 times daily). *Group 3:* (106 subjects) received oral ibuprofen (2 tablets, 4 times daily). *Group 4:* (20 subjects) received oral placebo (2 tablets, 4 times daily). *Group 5:* (19 subjects) received an unheated back wrap. All treatments were administered on 2 consecutive days.	All participants were assessed for pain relief, muscle stiffness, lateral trunk flexibility and by the Roland-Morris Disability Questionnaire. Efficacy was measured over the 2 treatment days and 2 follow-up days.	The study demonstrated that heat wrap, applied to the lumbar region, significantly improved pain relief, muscle stiffness, disability and lateral trunk flexion, compared with ibuprofen and acetaminophen.

Authors	Aim of study	Numbers	Methods	Assessment	Results
Nadler et al (2003)	To evaluate the efficacy of 8 h of continuous low-level heat wrap therapy for the treatment of acute non-specific low back pain.	219 subjects with acute non-specific low back pain were randomised into 4 groups.	Group 1: (95 subjects) received heat wrap to be worn for 8 h/day for 3 consecutive days. Group 2: (96 subjects) received oral placebo. Group 3: (12 subjects) received oral analgesia. Group 4: (16 subjects) received an unheated wrap.	All participants were assessed for pain relief, muscle stiffness, lateral trunk flexibility and by the Roland-Morris Disability Questionnaire.	A continuous low-level heat wrap was shown to provide significant therapeutic benefits in patients with acute non-specific low back pain, as indicated by increased pain relief and trunk flexibility, and it provided decreased muscle stiffness and disability when compared with placebo.
Robertson et al (2005)	To compare the effects on tissue extensibility (of the calf muscle) of shortwave diathermy (SWD) and hot packs.	24 subjects each received three different interventions.	1. SWD to the calf, at a 'comfortable warmth', for 15 min. 2. Hot pack to the calf for 15 min. 3. Remained resting on the plinth for 15 min (control).	Measurement of ankle dorsiflexion, using an inclinometer, pre- and post-intervention.	SWD increased ankle dorsiflexion by 1.8°, hot packs by 0.7° and control by 0.1°. The results indicate that SWD can significantly increase tissue extensibility.
Williams et al (1986)	To evaluate the use of superficial heat vs ice for the treatment of the rheumatoid arthritic (RA) shoulder.	18 subjects with RA shoulder were randomly allocated into two groups.	Group 1: (9 subjects) received hot packs for 20 min, followed by a 20 min exercise programme. Group 2: (9 subjects) received an ice pack for 20 min, followed by a 20 min exercise programme. Each subject received treatment 3 times a	Pain was measured using the McGill Pain Questionnaire. Range of movement (shoulder flexion and abduction) was measured using an electrogoniometer.	Both heat and ice reduced pain in the rheumatoid arthritic shoulder. A slightly greater range of movement was obtained using hot packs.

REFERENCES

Brosseau L, Robinson V, Pelland L et al 2002 Efficacy of thermotherapy for rheumatoid arthritis: a meta-analysis. Physical Therapy Reviews 7:5–15

French S D, Cameron M, Walker B F et al 2006 A Cochrane review of superficial heat or cold for low back pain. Spine 31:998–1006

Kauranen K, Vanharanta H 1997 Effects of hot and cold packs on motor performance of normal hands. Physiotherapy 83:340–344

Kitchen S 2002 Heat and cold: conduction methods. In: Kitchen S (ed) Electrotherapy: evidence-based practice, 11th edn. Churchill Livingstone, London, p 129–136

Mayer J M, Ralph L, Look M et al 2005 Treating acute low back pain with continuous low-level heat wrap therapy and/or exercise: a randomized controlled trial. Spine Journal 5:395–403

Michlovitz S, Hun L, Erasala G N et al 2004 Continuous low-level heat wrap therapy is effective for treating wrist pain. Archives of Physical Medicine and Rehabilitation 85:1409–1416

Nadler S F, Steiner D J, Erasala G N et al 2002 Continuous low-level heat wrap therapy provides more efficacy than ibuprofen and acetaminophen for acute low back pain. Spine 27:1012–1017

Nadler S F, Steiner D J, Erasala G N et al 2003 Continuous low-level heatwrap therapy for treating acute non-specific low back pain. Archives of Physical Medicine and Rehabilitation 84:329–334

Robertson V J, Ward A R, Jung P 2005 The effect of heat on tissue extensibility: a comparison of deep and superficial heating. Archives of Physical Medicine and Rehabilitation 86:819–825

Robertson V, Ward A, Low J et al 2006 Electrotherapy explained: principles and practice, 4th edn. Elsevier Science, Oxford

Williams J, Harvey J, Tannenbaum H 1986 Use of superficial heat versus ice for the rheumatoid arthritis shoulder: A pilot study. Physiotherapy Canada 38:8–13

CHAPTER 2

Paraffin wax bath

PRODUCTION

This is another form of conductive heating. Molten wax is a convenient method by which to apply heat to the extremities, as it contours well to the shape of the hands, feet, ankles and wrists. A small bath contains molten wax at a temperature of 42–52°C. Once applied to the hand, the wax solidifies to release a large amount of heat energy (latent heat), which is conducted into the tissues (Kitchen 2002, Robertson et al 2006).

EQUIPMENT

Molten wax bath (not shown)
Plastic wrap
Towel
Blanket
Hot and cold test tubes for skin sensation (thermal) testing
Thermometer.

⚠ Wax is highly flammable and therefore safety precautions should be taken not to mix with water and safety equipment should be at hand.

APPLICATION USING THE 'DIP AND WRAP' TECHNIQUE TO THE HAND

1. Ask the patient to wash and dry their hands (Fig. 2.2).
2. Position the patient, seated, beside the wax bath so they can easily reach into the wax bath.
3. Check that all jewellery has been removed and there are no cuts or infections on the hand.
4. Perform a skin sensation test on the area to be treated, ensuring palmar and dorsal surfaces are tested.
5. Check the temperature of the wax (42–52°C).

18 PRACTICAL ELECTROTHERAPY

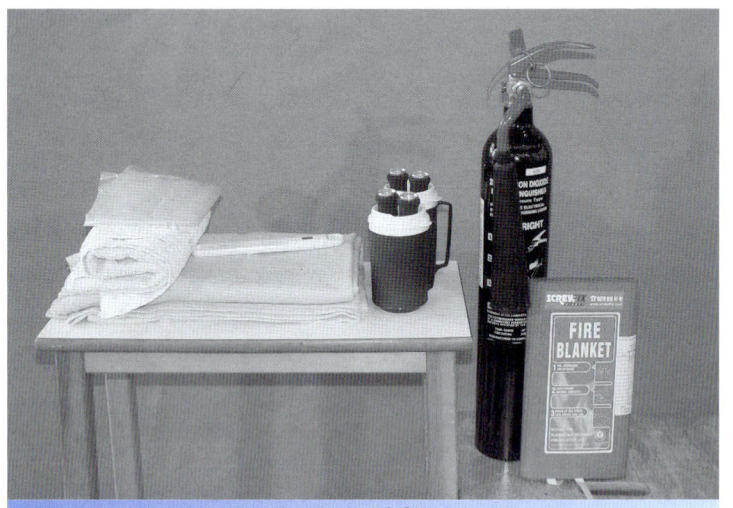

Figure 2.1 Equipment required for wax treatment.

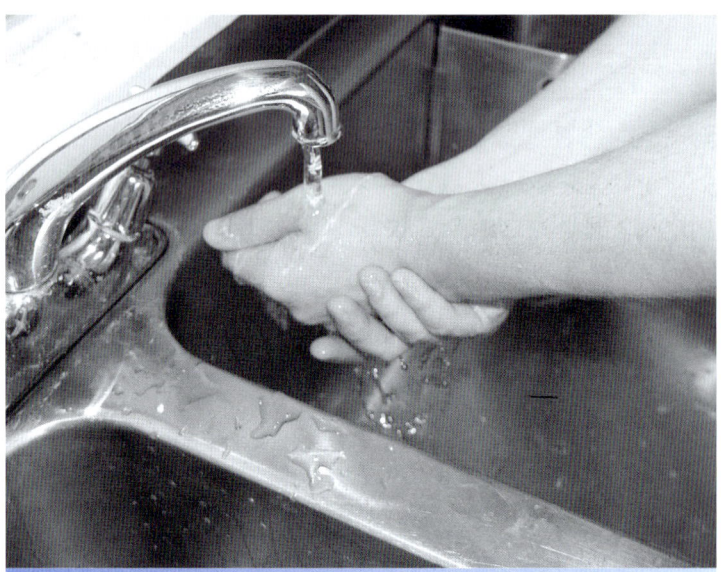

Figure 2.2 Wash and dry hands.

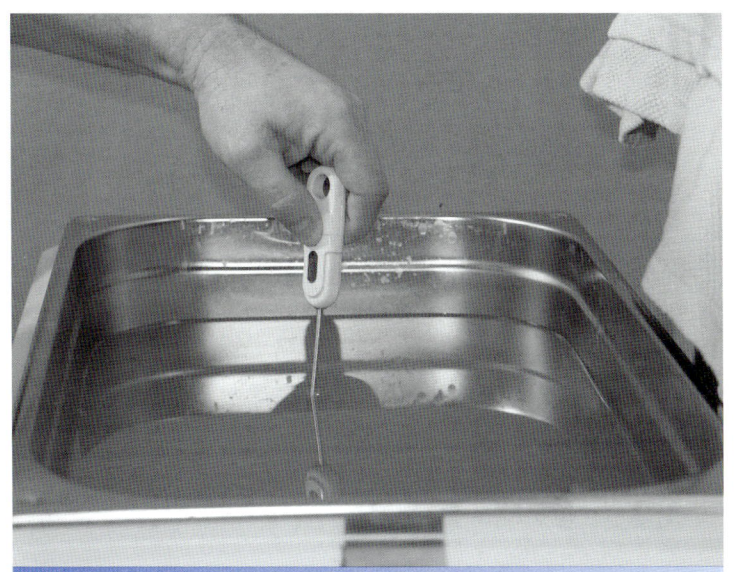

Figure 2.3 The temperature should be between 42°C and 52°C.

6. Explain the procedure to the patient and gain informed consent.
7. Prepare the patient with plastic wraps and towels ready for use.
8. Guide the patient's hand into the wax and hold for approximately 2–3 s (Fig. 2.4A,B).
9. Remove from the wax and allow the wax to solidify enough to stop dripping (Fig. 2.4C).
10. Repeat steps 8 and 9 until a thick coat of wax covers the hand – usually 6 or 7 dips. Do not leave the hand in the wax on the dip as the wax layers will not build up.
11. Wrap the hand in the plastic sheet, towel and blanket (Fig. 2.5A–C).
12. Set timer to the desired time, i.e. 15–20 min.
13. After treatment, inspect the area after removal of the wax.
14. Exercises can then be performed with the wax if desired (Fig. 2.6).
15. The wax is usually cleaned in a purifier and re-used.

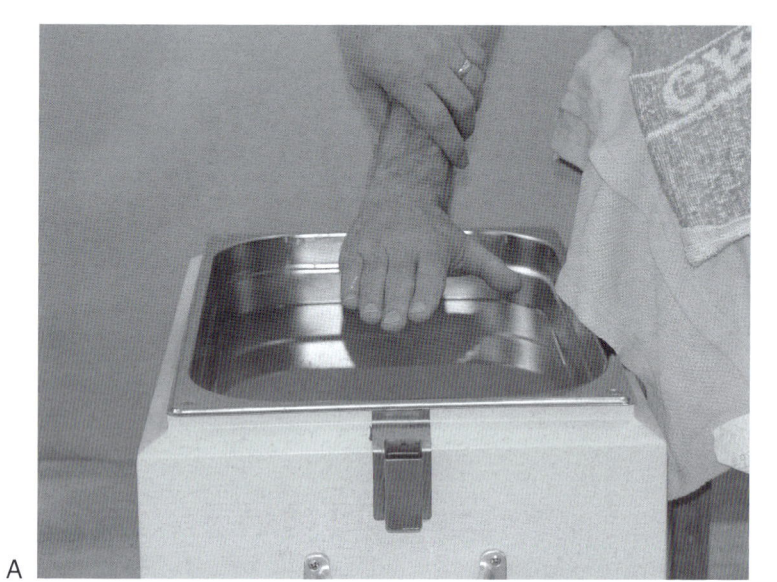

Figure 2.4 Dip and wrap technique. (A,B) Slowly guide the patient's hand into the wax and slowly out.

Paraffin wax bath

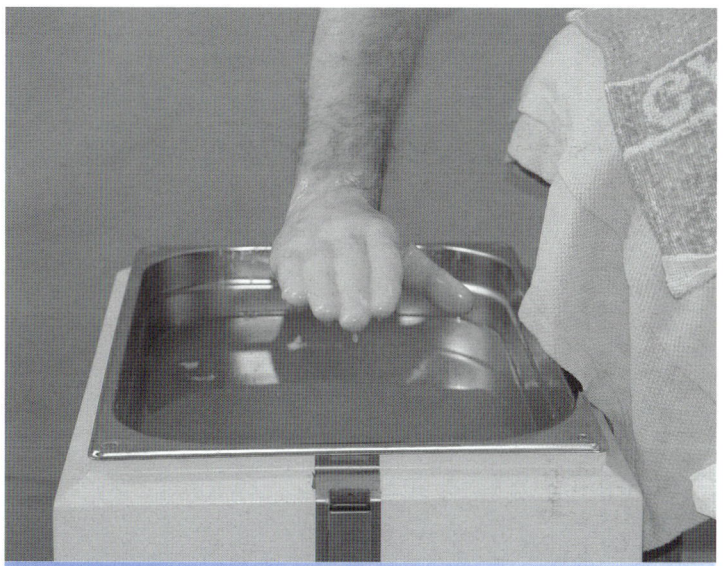

Figure 2.4, cont'd (C) Allow the wax to turn opaque before dipping into the wax to build up layers.

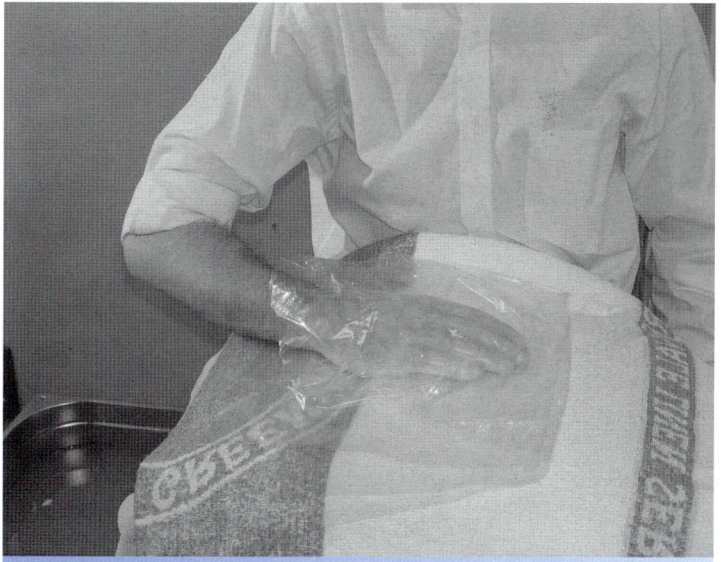

Figure 2.5 The stages of wrapping. (A–C) Once wrapped ensure that the limb is not left dependent as this may increase swelling in the area.

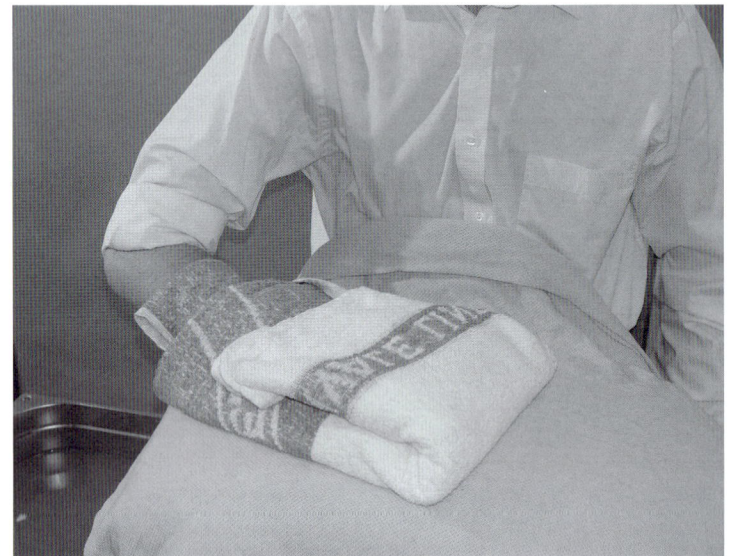

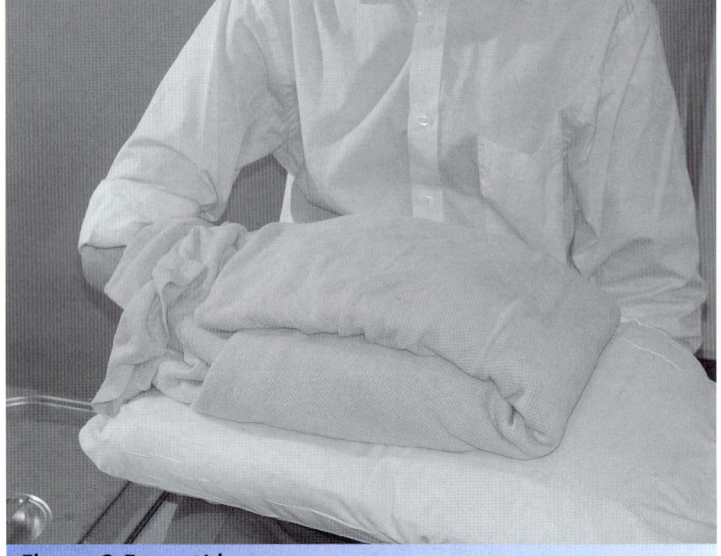

Figure 2.5, cont'd

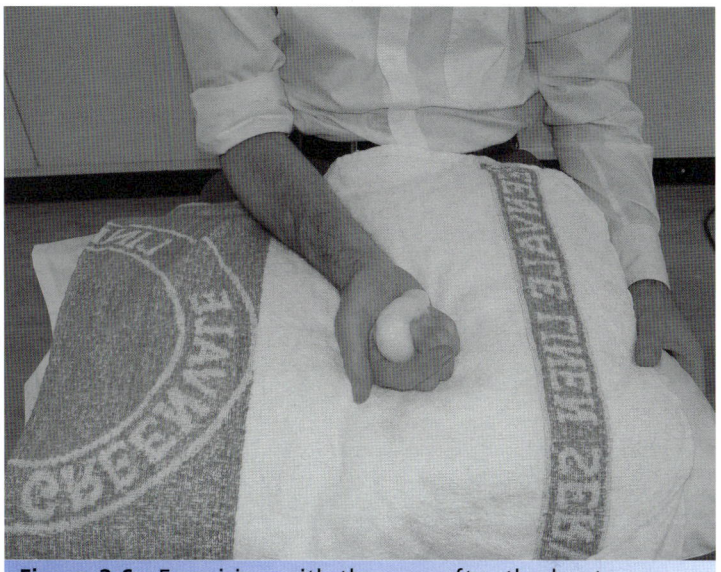

Figure 2.6 Exercising with the wax after the heat treatment.

Table 2.1 PHYSIOLOGICAL EFFECTS, USES AND CONTRAINDICATIONS

Physiological effect	Therapeutic uses	Contraindications/ precautions
↑ Metabolic activity	Encourage healing ↑ Metabolic rate ↑ Phagocytosis ↑ Oxygen release and use	Infections Acute inflammation Skin tumours Acute skin disease
↑ Blood supply	↑ Nutrient and O_2 supply ↓ Metabolites ↓ Chemical pain mediators	Impaired blood supply Drowsy patient Local bleeding
↑ Tissue fluid exchange	↓ Oedema	Acute trauma
Nerve stimulation	Sensory/thermal: ↓ Pain Golgi tendon inhibition: ↓ Muscle spasm	Defective sensation
↓ Viscosity	↓ Peripheral resistance Synovial fluid: ↑ Joint range	Defective blood pressure regulation
↑ Extensibility of collagen	Precursor to stretching	

See also Robertson et al (2006).

Notes

Paraffin wax bath

Treatment record

Table 2.2 **OBSERVATIONAL/REFLECTIVE CHECKLIST**

	Observation	Y/N	Comments
Introduction	Did the therapist introduce him/herself?	☐	☐
	Was an explanation of the procedure given?	☐	☐
	Was the explanation clear and succinct?	☐	☐
	Were the possible dangers highlighted?	☐	☐
	Was consent obtained?	☐	☐
Comfort and safety	Was the patient comfortable?	☐	☐
	Was the therapist's posture compromised?	☐	☐
	Was the position safe for both parties?	☐	☐
	Was the modality applied with due care and attention?	☐	☐
Technique	Were the contraindications checked?	☐	☐
	Were the appropriate tests performed prior to treatment?	☐	☐
	Was an explanation of the physiological effects of the technique offered to the patient?	☐	☐
	Was this explanation accurate?	☐	☐
	Was the technique/modality applied correctly?	☐	☐
	Were the correct times and settings used?	☐	☐
	Was the skin checked after the treatment for adverse effects?	☐	☐

Table 2.3 SUMMARY OF STUDIES INVESTIGATING THE EFFECTIVENESS OF HEAT TREATMENTS – WAX

Authors	Aim of study	Numbers	Methods	Assessment	Results
Ayling & Marks (2000)	This paper summarises the randomised controlled trials evaluating the effects of paraffin wax for rheumatoid arthritis (RA). The authors conclude by stating that their data suggest there may be some benefit, with few side-effects, in the application of paraffin wax to the hands of people with non-acute RA, prior to exercise. Also, the data are insufficient and preclude any definitive conclusions concerning the efficacy of paraffin wax for treating painful hand arthritis.				
Brosseau et al (2002)	The reviewers conclude that thermotherapy (hot packs, ice packs, paraffin wax baths and faradic baths) can be used as a palliative therapy, or as an adjunct therapy combined with exercise for rheumatoid arthritic patients, especially wax baths in the treatment of arthritic hands. They also said that the conclusions are limited by methodological considerations, such as the poor quality of trials.				
Buljina et al (2001)	To evaluate the effectiveness of physical therapy (wax baths or ice massage, thermal baths, faradic hand baths and exercise therapy) for rheumatoid arthritis (RA) in the hands.	100 patients with RA hands were randomly assigned to a treatment group or control group (on the waiting list for 4 weeks).	*The Treatment Group*: (50 subjects) received a daily physical therapy programme (thermal bath for 20 min, faradic hand baths for 15 min, wax baths for 20 min, and an individual exercise programme for 20–30 min) for 3 weeks (15 treatments). *The Control Group*: (50 subjects) remained on the waiting list for 1 month.	All participants were assessed at the commencement of the study and at the end of the 3-week study period. The patient's assessment consisted of the erythrocyte sedimentation rate (ESR), pain intensity, joint tenderness, palmar tip-to-tip and key pinch finger strength, finger range of movement and activities of daily living (ADL).	The treatment group demonstrated a significant reduction in pain intensity and joint tenderness, and a significant increase in hand strength, range of movement and ADL.

PRACTICAL ELECTROTHERAPY

Authors	Aim of study	Numbers	Methods	Assessment	Results
Dellhag et al (1992)	To evaluate the effects in rheumatoid arthritic (RA) patients of active hand exercises and wax bath treatment alone and in combination in a randomised controlled trial.	52 patients with RA were randomly assigned to one of four groups.	Group 1: (13 subjects) received wax bath treatment followed by active hand exercises. Group 2: (11 subjects) received active exercises only. Group 3: (15 subjects) received wax bath treatment only. Group 4: (13 subjects) were the control group. Treatment was given 3 times a week for 4 weeks.	The outcome measurements assessed were: range of movement (ROM), grip function, grip strength, pain and stiffness.	Wax bath and active hand exercises resulted in a significant improvement in ROM and grip strength. Active hand exercises alone reduced stiffness and pain and increased ROM. Wax bath treatment alone had no significant effect.
Hawkes et al (1986)	To compare three different physiotherapy treatments for rheumatoid arthritis of the hands.	30 patients with rheumatoid arthritis of the hands were assigned to three groups.	Group 1: (10 subjects) received wax (20 min) treatment and exercises, 5 days a week for 3 weeks. Group 2: (10 subjects) received ultrasound in a water bath (3 MHz, constant, intensity of 0.25 W/cm^2 for 3 min to palmar and 3 min to dorsal aspect of each hand) and exercises, 5 days a week for 3 weeks.	Patients were assessed prior to treatment and at weeks 1, 2 and 3 of the treatment. The following assessments were performed: grip strength using a sphygmomanometer cuff, joint size using a specialised tape measure, visual	All outcome measures showed significant improvement by the end of the third week of treatment in all treatment groups.

Authors	Aim of study	Numbers	Methods	Assessment	Results
			Group 3: (10 subjects) received ultrasound (parameters as above), faradic baths (standard technique) for 15 min and exercises, 5 days a week for 3 weeks.	analogue scale (VAS) for pain, articular index score for pain/tenderness, range of movement, timed task and a checklist of activities.	
Sandqvist et al (2004)	To investigate the effects of treatment with paraffin wax baths in patients with systemic sclerosis (scleroderma).	17 patients with scleroderma had one hand treated with wax and the other acted as a control.	Each participant received instruction on how to apply the wax at home. They dipped their selected hand 5–6 times into the wax bath, wrapped it in a quilt mitten and rested for 10 min. Hand exercises were performed on both hands immediately after the wax treatment. This regime was carried out daily for 1 month. The other hand acted as the control.	Patients were assessed before treatment and after 1 month of treatment, concerning hand joint mobility, grip force, and perceived pain, stiffness and skin elasticity.	After 1 month of treatment, finger flexion and extension, thumb abduction, wrist flexion, stiffness and skin elasticity had significantly improved in the wax-treated hand compared with the baseline values ($p < 0.05$).

REFERENCES

Ayling J, Marks R 2000 Efficacy of paraffin wax baths for rheumatoid arthritic hands. Physiotherapy 86:190–201

Brosseau L, Robinson V, Pelland L et al 2002 Efficacy of thermotherapy for rheumatoid arthritis: a meta-analysis. Physical Therapy Reviews 7:5–15

Buljina A I, Taljanovic M S, Avdic D M et al 2001 Physical and exercise therapy for treatment of the rheumatoid hand. Arthritis Care and Research 45:392–397

Dellhag B, Wollersjö I, Bjelle A 1992 Effect of active hand exercise and wax bath treatment in rheumatoid arthritis patients. Arthritis Care and Research 5:87–91

Hawkes J, Care G, Dixon J S et al 1986 A comparison of three different physiotherapy treatments for rheumatoid arthritis of the hands. Physiotherapy Practice 2:155–160

Kitchen S 2002 Heat and cold: conduction methods. In: Kitchen S (ed) Electrotherapy: evidence-based practice, 11th edn. Churchill Livingstone, London, p 129–136

Robertson V, Ward A, Low J et al 2006 Electrotherapy explained: principles and practice, 4th edn. Elsevier Science, Oxford

Sandqvist G, Åkesson A, Eklund M 2004 Evaluation of paraffin bath treatment in patients with systemic sclerosis. Disability and Rehabilitation 26:981–987

CHAPTER 3

Shortwave diathermy

PRODUCTION

The shortwave diathermy (SWD) machine produces an alternating current with a frequency of 27.12 MHz. This current is produced by a sine-wave generator within the oscillatory circuit. The oscillatory circuit transfers this high-frequency current to the patient or resonator circuit, by means of electromagnetic induction. This involves a coil in each circuit being placed close together, forming a transformer, so that the magnetic field generated by the oscillator circuit induces a current in the resonator circuit. The current oscillating between the two electrodes (also known as capacitors or condensers) does so at a frequency of 27.12 MHz. Energy will be effectively transferred if the two are in tune (*c.f.* tuning a radio). Most modern SWD machines have an automatic tuning mechanism.

The two capacitors consist of two metal plates separated by an insulator (dielectric). They are able to store an electric charge. As the current oscillates backwards and forwards between the two capacitors (at 27 million times/s), each will hold, alternately, a positive and negative charge. As the capacitor plates are given opposite electrical charges, electric lines of force will concentrate between the plates. There is therefore an electric field between the capacitors. The patient is part of this resonator circuit (Fig. 3.1).

This causes heating in the tissues due to ionic motion, dipole rotation and molecular distortion (Robertson et al 2006, Scott 2002).

PRACTICAL ELECTROTHERAPY

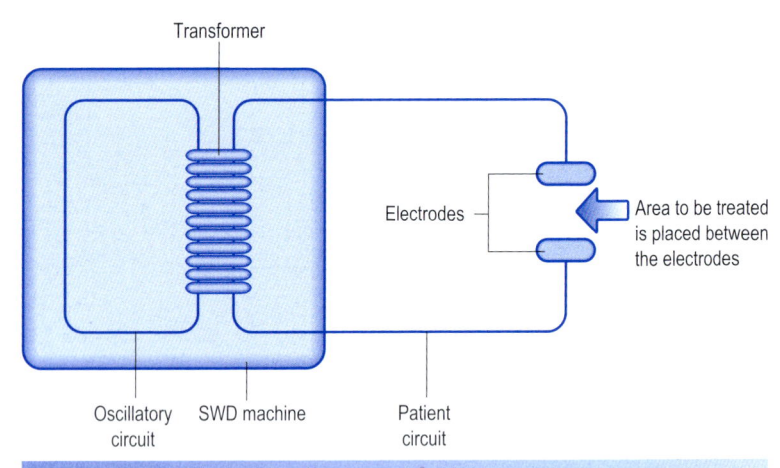

Figure 3.1 Schematic diagram of SWD.

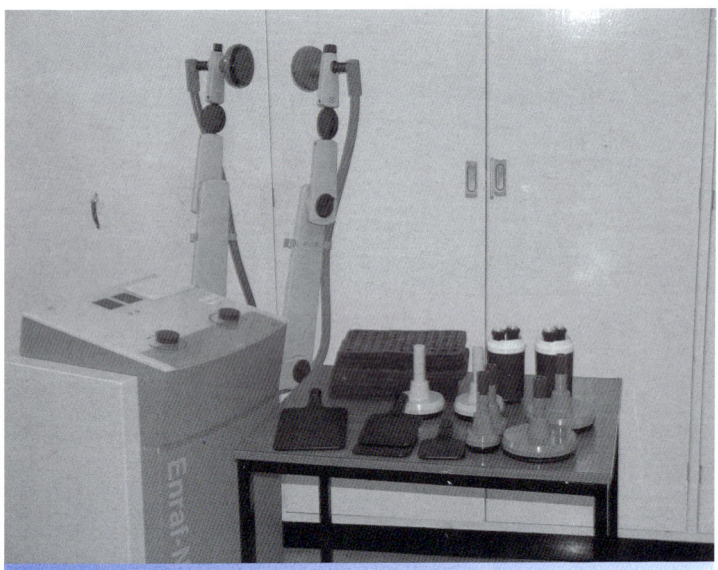

Figure 3.2 SWD machine with various electrodes.

Shortwave diathermy

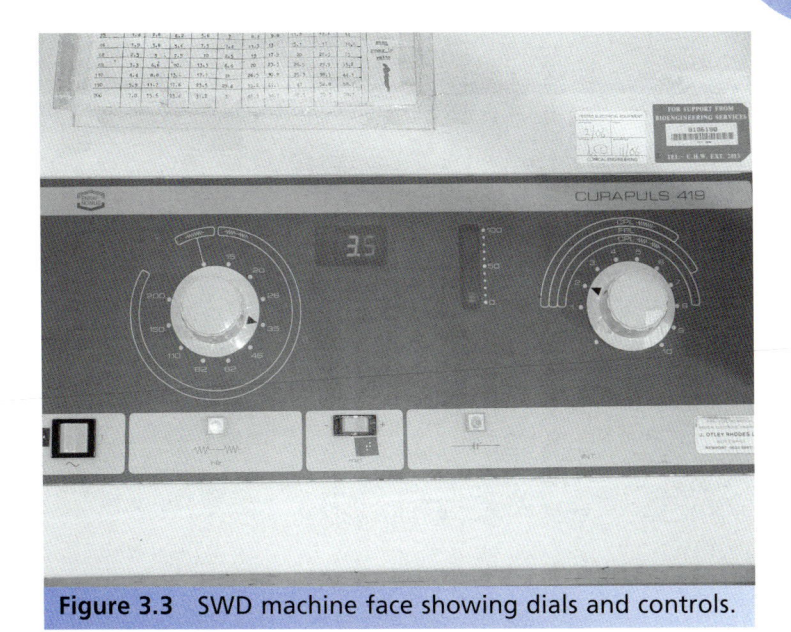

Figure 3.3 SWD machine face showing dials and controls.

APPLICATION, CONTRAPLANAR TO THE SHOULDER

1. Select electrodes slightly larger than the area to be treated. Connect them to the machine and plug the machine into the wall socket.
2. For SWD the freguency dial (the left dial in Fig. 3.3) should be set to continuous.
3. Test the machine is working by placing your hand or a neon tube between the electrodes. Slowly turn up the intensity until you feel a gentle warmth on your hand or the neon tube begins to glow (Fig. 3.4A,B).
4. Position the patient as in Figure 3.5 on a chair with the arm supported on a table, resting on a pillow. Ensure that when positioning the patient the arm is away from the side so that sweat does not build up in the axilla, as water will concentrate the field and may cause a burn. This is the same for any area of the body, therefore make sure that limbs are placed in a position so that there is no skin to skin contact.
5. Perform a skin sensation test to the area to be treated.
6. Dry the area with a towel.
7. Explain the procedure to the patient and re-check for any contraindications and remove all metal jewellery from the area.
8. Gain informed consent.

34 PRACTICAL ELECTROTHERAPY

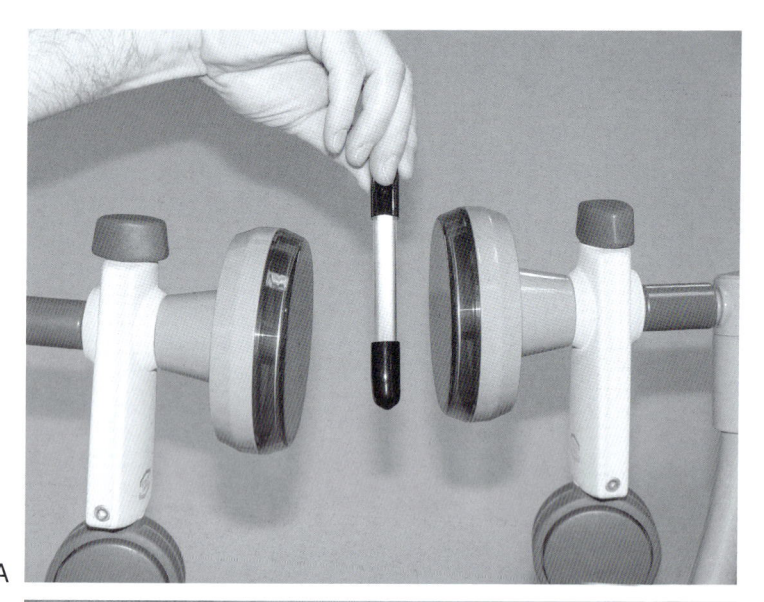

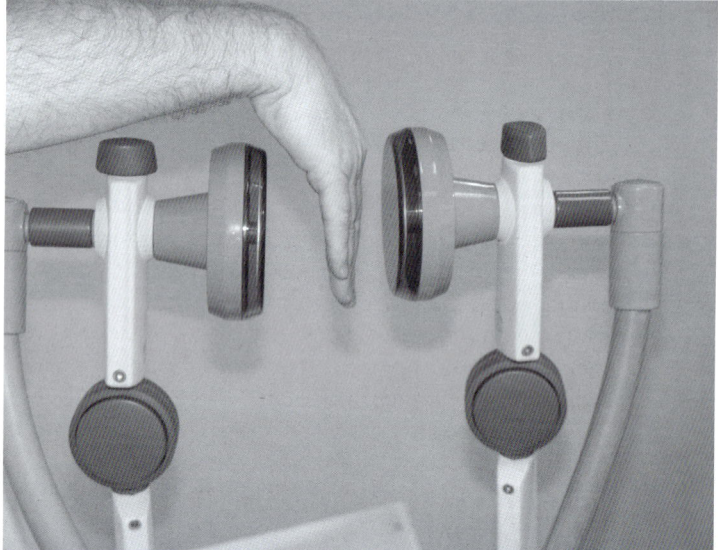

Figure 3.4 Testing the machine with (A) a neon tube or (B) with your hand. Place the tube or your hand between the electrodes and then turn on the machine. Gradually turn up the intensity until the tube glows or you feel a gentle warmth on both sides of your hand. Turn the machine off before removing your hand or the tube.

Shortwave diathermy

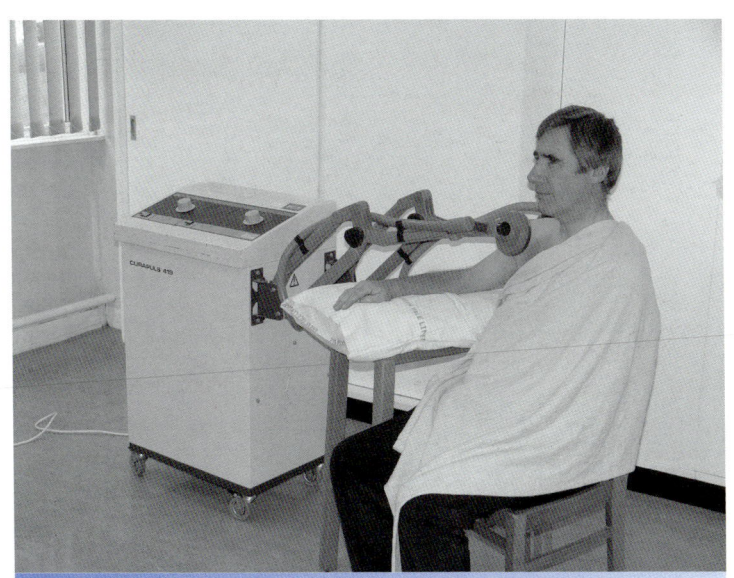

Figure 3.5 SWD application to the right shoulder.

9. Mark the position of the joint line (from the coracoid process, 1 cm laterally) (Fig. 3.6).
10. Position the machine as in Figure 3.6, parallel with the arm.
11. Position the electrodes parallel and about 2–4 cm away from the skin, the centre being in line with the centre of the joint line marked (Fig. 3.6).
12. Ensure all the cables and leads are a safe distance from the patient.
13. Turn the machine on; set the time to 10, 15 or 20 min and increase the intensity until the mild, comfortable warmth is felt. The patient is warned about the possibility of a burn.
14. Do not leave the area. You are instantly available to turn down the machine if the application becomes hot. The patient should not read or fall asleep during the treatment.
15. At the end of the treatment, check the skin for any adverse reactions.

VARIATIONS IN SET-UP

The shape and size of the field will be determined by the orientation of the electrodes relative to each other and on what is placed between them (see Fig. 3.9).

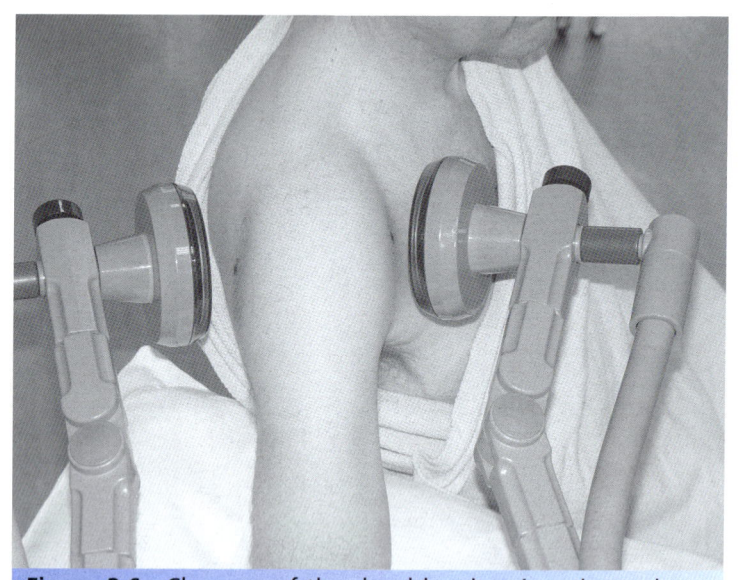

Figure 3.6 Close-up of the shoulder showing electrode positioning around the centre of the joint (marked in pen).

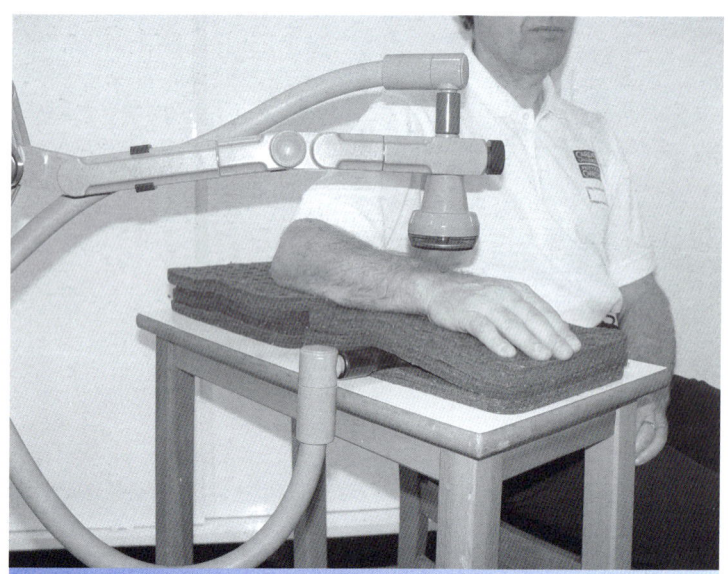

Figure 3.7 SWD (contraplanar) to the wrist. Set-up for wrist, using a small condenser electrode and a small malleable electrode. (May use medium electrodes if the wrist is larger.) The elbow is fully supported on three felt spacers. The malleable electrode is placed on top of a felt spacer, with two further felt spacers on top. This gives the required spacing necessary for a safe treatment.

Shortwave diathermy

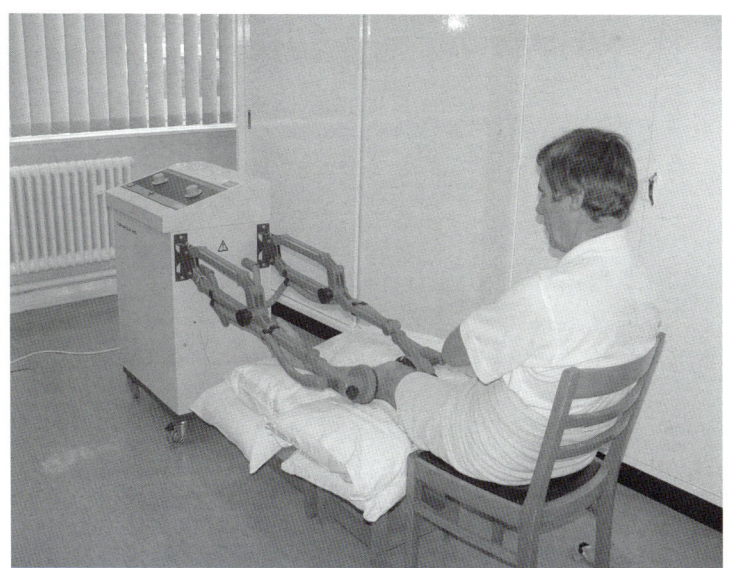

Figure 3.8 SWD (contraplanar) to the knee. The patient sits on a wooden chair, leg comfortably resting on pillows, which are positioned on wooden stools. The pillows do not have a plastic covering. Two medium size electrodes are placed on either side of the knee joint, parallel to the skin. Felt spacers may be required to protect the foot from the leads. When treating the ankle joint, medium or small electrodes may be used, depending on the size of the joint. These should be placed parallel to the ankle joint, with a spacing of approximately 4 cm. This distance is required to prevent a concentration of the field at the bony malleoli.

Physiological effects, therapeutic uses and contraindications

Below is the table (Table 3.1) that can also be seen in the other modalities within this heating and cooling section. This is because they are common to all heating modalities.

As SWD is a more complex form of heating compared with simple conduction methods, and electromagnetic fields are involved, it has specific precautions and contraindications. These specific precautions and contraindications for SWD are listed below.

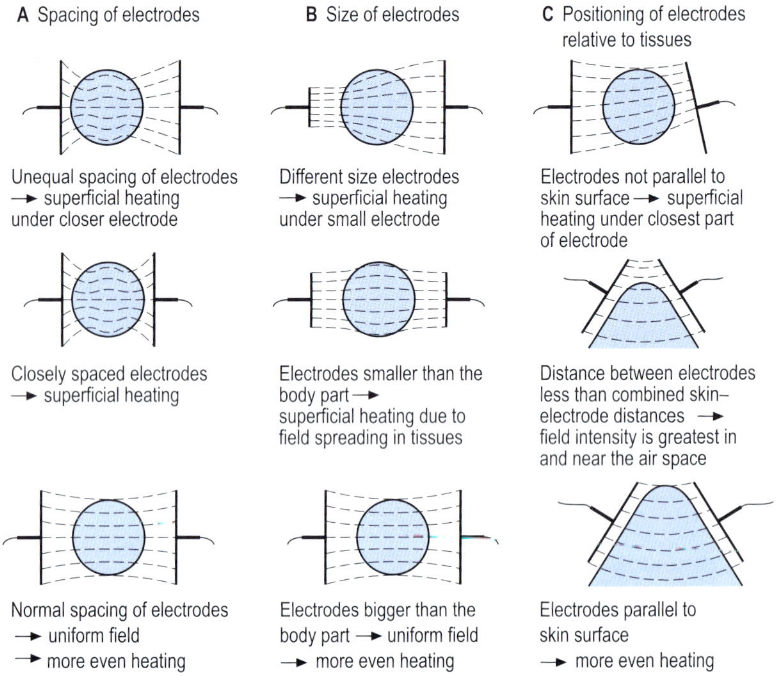

PRACTICAL ELECTROTHERAPY

Figure 3.9 The effect of positioning electrodes on the electric field through tissues using a contraplanar technique (from Robertson et al 2006, with permission).

A Spacing of electrodes

Unequal spacing of electrodes → superficial heating under closer electrode

Closely spaced electrodes → superficial heating

Normal spacing of electrodes → uniform field → more even heating

B Size of electrodes

Different size electrodes → superficial heating under small electrode

Electrodes smaller than the body part → superficial heating due to field spreading in tissues

Electrodes bigger than the body part → uniform field → more even heating

C Positioning of electrodes relative to tissues

Electrodes not parallel to skin surface → superficial heating under closest part of electrode

Distance between electrodes less than combined skin–electrode distances → field intensity is greatest in and near the air space

Electrodes parallel to skin surface → more even heating

Dangers
Burns
Metal implants
Cardiac pacemakers
Synthetic material
Obese patients
Treatment over the uterus during pregnancy
Distance from machine
Implanted slow-release hormone capsule.

Specific contraindications and precautions
Metal in the area, including implants
Cardiac pacemaker
Haemorrhagic conditions
Ischaemic conditions

Table 3.1 *PHYSIOLOGICAL EFFECTS AND CONTRAINDICATIONS*

Physiological effect	Therapeutic uses	Contraindications/ precautions
↑ Metabolic activity	Encourage healing ↑ Metabolic rate ↑ Phagocytosis ↑ Oxygen release and use	Infections Acute inflammation Skin tumours Acute skin disease
↑ Blood supply	↑ Nutrient and O_2 supply ↓ Metabolites ↓ Chemical pain mediators	Impaired blood supply Drowsy patient Deep X-ray therapy Local bleeding
↑ Tissue fluid exchange	↓ Oedema	
Nerve stimulation	Sensory/thermal: ↓ Pain Golgi tendon inhibition: ↓ Muscle spasm	
↓ Viscosity	↓ Peripheral resistance Synovial fluid: ↑ Joint range	Defective blood pressure regulation
↑ Extensibility of collagen	Precursor to stretching	

Malignant tumours
Active TB
Pregnancy
Post-venous thrombosis
Impaired thermal sensation
When patient is pyrexic
After deep X-ray therapy (devitalised skin)
Patient who is unable to stay still or cooperate.

Students are directed specifically to Robertson et al (2006), Scott (2002) and to the Chartered Society of Physiotherapy (CSP) guidelines (1997).

Notes

Shortwave diathermy

Treatment record

Table 3.2 *OBSERVATIONAL/REFLECTIVE CHECKLIST*

	Observation	Y/N	Comments
Introduction	Did the therapist introduce him/herself?	☐	☐
	Was an explanation of the procedure given?	☐	☐
	Was the explanation clear and succinct?	☐	☐
	Were the possible dangers highlighted?	☐	☐
	Was consent obtained?	☐	☐
Comfort and safety	Was the patient comfortable?	☐	☐
	Was the therapist's posture compromised?	☐	☐
	Was the position safe for both parties?	☐	☐
	Was the modality applied with due care and attention?	☐	☐
Technique	Were the contraindications checked?	☐	☐
	Were the appropriate tests performed prior to treatment?	☐	☐
	Was an explanation of the physiological effects of the technique offered to the patient?	☐	☐
	Was this explanation accurate?	☐	☐
	Was the technique/modality applied correctly?	☐	☐
	Were the correct times and settings used?	☐	☐
	Was the skin checked after the treatment for adverse effects?	☐	☐

Table 3.3 SUMMARY OF STUDIES INVESTIGATING THE EFFECTIVENESS OF SHORTWAVE DIATHERMY (SWD)

Authors	Aim of study	Numbers	Methods	Assessment	Results
Chartered Society of Physiotherapy (CSP) (1997)	This fact sheet, written by the CSP, considers the safe and efficacious practice of shortwave diathermy (SWD) and pulsed shortwave diathermy (PSWD).		Recent research suggests that with modern SWD/PSWD machines, the field strength beyond 1 m should fall below the safe exposure limits. 1 m is therefore the minimum recommended distance between a SWD/PSWD and a member of staff, another patient or other electrical equipment. During treatment, CSP members should stay outside the 1 m zone.		

Shortwave diathermy 43

Authors	Aim of study	Numbers	Methods	Assessment	Results
Gray et al (1995)	To evaluate and compare the effects of four different electrotherapeutic modalities, namely shortwave diathermy, megapulse (pulsed shortwave diathermy), ultrasound and laser therapy on patients with temporo-mandibular pain dysfunction (TMPDS).	139 patients with TMPDS were randomly allocated into one of five groups.	*Group 1:* (27 subjects) received shortwave diathermy at a mild setting for 10 min. *Group 2:* (27 subjects) received megapulse (pulsed shortwave) (pulse frequency 100 Hz, pulse duration 60 µs) for 20 min. *Group 3:* (30 subjects) received ultrasound (3 MHz, pulsed 2:1, intensity of 0.25 W/cm^2) for 2 min. *Group 4:* (29 subjects) received laser therapy (wavelength 904 nm, dosage of 4 J/cm^2) for 3 min. *Group 5:* (26 subjects) received placebo treatment with one of the above modalities. All participants received treatment 3 times a week for 4 weeks.	Assessment of improvement was made objectively on the basis of a total symptom profile. Those symptoms recorded pre- and post-treatment were muscle tenderness, joint sounds and joint tenderness on direct palpation. Range of movement (ROM) was measured and the subjective improvement was recorded on the basis of the patients' report on their overall state (worse, unchanged, variable, much better or cured).	At the time of the first review, 7 days after the completion of treatment, there was no significant difference in the success rate between any of the treatment groups or between the treated and placebo groups. At the final review, at 3 months, a definite and significant difference between the treated and placebo groups had emerged.

Authors	Aim of study	Numbers	Methods	Assessment	Results
Jan et al (2006)	To investigate whether repetitive shortwave diathermy (SWD) could reduce synovitis in patients with osteoarthritis (OA) of the knee and to examine the relationship between synovial thickness and pain index.	30 patients, with 44 OA knees were divided into three groups.	*Group 1*: (11 patients/14 knees) received SWD, at a 'mild but pleasant sensation of heat' for 20 min. *Group 2*: (10 patients/14 knees) received SWD and NSAIDs. *Group 3*: (9 patients/16 knees) acted as a control (no treatment). Each participant received 30 treatments over 8 weeks.	Every participant was assessed by ultrasonographic imaging, performed at the initial and three follow-up sessions. Pain was assessed using the visual analogue scale (VAS), before and after each treatment.	The results suggest that a decrease in synovial sac thickness and knee pain is induced with a series of SWD treatments.

Authors	Aim of study	Numbers	Methods	Assessment	Results
Kitchen & Partridge (1992)	This is an extensive paper discussing the physical effects of continuous and pulsed shortwave diathermy and their physiological effects, with regard to the thermal and athermal mechanisms. The efficacy of both continuous and pulsed shortwave diathermy is examined through the use of both experimental models (animal studies) and clinical trials. Experimental studies have been undertaken on soft tissues and joints, whereas clinical trials have been undertaken on soft tissues, joint studies and pain relief. Hazards of shortwave diathermy have been identified.				
Marks et al (1999)	This is a review paper examining the efficacy of shortwave diathermy (SWD) for alleviating the main symptoms of OA of the knee.	11 relevant trials were included in the review.	The authors undertook a systematic search of literature. This revealed 11 studies, non-randomised comparative and randomised controlled trials (RCTs), which were reviewed by the authors.		The authors conclude that further controlled studies are essential to establish whether either continuous or pulsed SWD is efficacious for treating patients with OA of the knee.
Pope et al (1995)	To assess the current clinical use of electrotherapeutic modalities in the NHS in England.		Pulsed shortwave diathermy (PSWD) and shortwave diathermy (SWD) units were widely owned and frequently used. A total of 209 respondents owned PSWD units and only six respondents did not use this modality. Out of 190 respondents, over two-thirds (132) used PSWD 2–3 times/day and a further 20 respondents used PSWD daily. A total of 196 respondents owned SWD units and 68 respondents did not use this modality. Out of 113 respondents, only 22 used SWD 2–3 times/day and a further 12 respondents used SWD daily.		

Authors	Aim of study	Numbers	Methods	Assessment	Results
Quirk et al (1985)	To evaluate the effects of interferential therapy (IFT), shortwave diathermy and exercises in the treatment of OA of the knee.	38 patients with OA of the knee were randomly allocated to three groups.	*Group 1:* (12 subjects) received IFT (suction electrodes, frequency 0–100 Hz for 10 min and 130 Hz for 5 min) and exercises (straight leg raise (SLR) × 30, twice daily). *Group 2:* (12 subjects) received shortwave diathermy (condenser field method for 20 min) and exercises. *Group 3:* (14 subjects) received exercises only and were told to continue to the end of the trial.	Patients were assessed before, on completion of their course of treatment and 3–6 months following completion of their treatment. Range of movement, walking distance, and maximum knee girth were assessed. Pain, using the visual analogue scale (VAS), and function were also assessed.	At the end of the treatment, there was a significant improvement in the mean pain scores and overall clinical condition of all three groups.

Authors	Aim of study	Numbers	Methods	Assessment	Results
Robertson et al (2005)	To compare the effects on tissue extensibility (of the calf muscle) of SWD and hot packs.	24 subjects, each received three different interventions.	1. SWD to the calf, at a 'comfortable warmth', for 15 min. 2. Hot pack to the calf for 15 min. 3. Remained resting on the plinth for 15 min (control).	Measurement of ankle dorsiflexion, using an inclinometer, pre- and post-intervention.	SWD increased ankle dorsiflexion by 1.8°, hot packs by 0.7° and control by 0.1°. The results indicate that SWD can significantly increase tissue extensibility.
Shields et al (2002)	To establish the current clinical and safety practices during continuous (CSWD) and pulsed (PSWD) SWD application in Ireland.	83 questionnaires.	Questionnaires were sent to Irish-based physiotherapy departments using SWD. (75% return).		PSWD was the preferred mode. CSWD was rated effective for treating chronic OA, polyarthritis, non-specific arthrosis, haematomas, acute arthritis, sinusitis and RA. There were questions concerning safety practices.

Authors	Aim of study	Numbers	Methods	Assessment	Results
Shields et al (2004)	To investigate the documented evidence for the contraindications to shortwave diathermy (SWD) and to determine the level of agreement among senior physiotherapists.	116 questionnaires distributed to Irish physiotherapists.	The physiotherapists were asked to categorise 35 symptoms or conditions as either 'always', 'sometimes', or 'never' contraindicated, or 'don't know' whether contraindicated for both continuous and pulsed shortwave diathermy.	The data were analysed using descriptive statistics.	There was a 75% response rate. Over 90% agreement was found among respondents for traditional contraindications to both continuous shortwave diathermy (metal implants, pacemakers, malignancy, tuberculous joints, over the eyes) and pulsed shortwave diathermy (malignancy and pacemakers). The authors concluded that there was an overall lack of research-based evidence regarding most contraindications to treatment.

Authors	Aim of study	Numbers	Methods	Assessment	Results
Shields et al (2005)	To investigate how physiotherapists perceive the risk exposure to stray radiofrequency radiation (electromagnetic fields) in the physiotherapy department, in particular the use of shortwave diathermy.	225 questionnaires were sent to physios working in hospital-based physiotherapy departments.	The questionnaire consisted of four sections. Section 1 consisted of background data questions. Section 2 required respondents to rate their perception of risk for 23 items. Section 3 asked respondents to rate the level of health consequences they perceived would occur from exposure to 22 of the 23 risk items. In section 4, respondents were asked how often they would be able to protect themselves from exposure to 15 risks.	Microsoft Access and SPSS statistical packages were used for data analysis.	Of the 225 questionnaires delivered, 203 were completed (90.2%). Respondents were found to perceive exposure to electromagnetic fields (EMFs) as low risk. The respondents also felt they could often protect themselves from the risk of stray EMFs. The authors concluded that respondents were complacent about the dangers involved and therefore few safety measures were taken.

REFERENCES

Chartered Society of Physiotherapy (CSP) 1997 Employment relations and union services: health and safety – safe practice with electrotherapy (shortwave therapies). CSP, London. Online. Available: www.csp.org.uk

Gray R J, Quayle A A, Hall C A et al 1995 Temporomandibular pain dysfunction: can electrotherapy help? Physiotherapy 81:47–51

Jan M H, Chai H M, Lin Y F et al 2006 Effects of repetitive shortwave diathermy for reducing synovitis in patients with knee osteoarthritis: an ultrasonographic study. Physical Therapy 82:236–244

Kitchen S, Partridge C 1992 Review of shortwave diathermy continuous and pulsed patterns. Physiotherapy 78:243–252

Marks R, Ghassemi M, Duarte R et al 1999 A review of the literature on shortwave diathermy as applied to osteo-arthritis of the knee. Physiotherapy 85:304–316

Pope G D, Mockett S P, Wright J P 1995 A survey of electrotherapy modalities: ownership and use in the NHS in England. Physiotherapy 81:82–91

Quirk A S, Newman R J, Newman K J 1985 An evaluation of interferential therapy, shortwave diathermy and exercise in the treatment of osteoarthrosis of the knee. Physiotherapy 71:55–57

Robertson V J, Ward A R, Jung P 2005 The effect of heat on tissue extensibility: a comparison of deep and superficial heating. Archives of Physical Medicine and Rehabilitation 86:819–825

Robertson V, Ward A, Low J et al 2006 Electrotherapy explained: principles and practice, 4th edn. Elsevier Science, Oxford

Scott S 2002 Part 1 – Short-wave diathermy. In: Kitchen S (ed) Electrotherapy: evidence-based practice, 11th edn. Churchill Livingstone, London, p 145–165

Shields N, Gormley J, O'Hare N 2002 Short-wave diathermy: current clinical and safety practices. Physiotherapy Research International 7:191–202

Shields N, O'Hare N, Gormley J 2004 Contra-indications to shortwave diathermy: survey of Irish physiotherapists. Physiotherapy 90:42–53

Shields N, Gormley J, O'Hare N 2005 Physiotherapists' perception of risk from electromagnetic fields. Advances in Physiotherapy 7:170–175

CHAPTER 4

Ice/cold packs (cryotherapy)

PRODUCTION

When an ice pack or cold pack is applied to the skin, heat is conducted from the area of high temperature to that of a lower temperature, i.e. from the skin to the ice. This energy in the form of heat is used to change the ice from a solid to a liquid, which requires a considerable amount of energy (latent heat of fusion of ice). There are several methods for applying ice. Below is a description of an ice pack to the knee (see also Robertson et al 2006, Kitchen 2002).

ICE PACK APPLICATION TO THE KNEE

1. The patient is positioned in a half-lying position.
2. The knee is exposed and put in a comfortable position.
3. A gutter of polythene is placed under the knee.
4. Perform a skin sensation (thermal) test to the area to be treated.
5. Explain the procedure to the patient and re-check any contraindications.
6. Gain informed consent from the patient.
7. Prepare the tray (see Fig 4.1).
8. Apply oil to the area to be treated. This helps to reduce the chance of an ice burn.
9. Place the ice pack over the knee and set the timer for 20–30 min (Fig. 4.2).
10. Excess water should run down the gutter into the bath, not onto the floor (Fig. 4.2).
11. Inspect the skin after several minutes to check the skin reaction (Fig. 4.3).
12. The ice pack is left on for 20–30 min (CSP 1998).
13. After treatment, check the area for any adverse reactions.

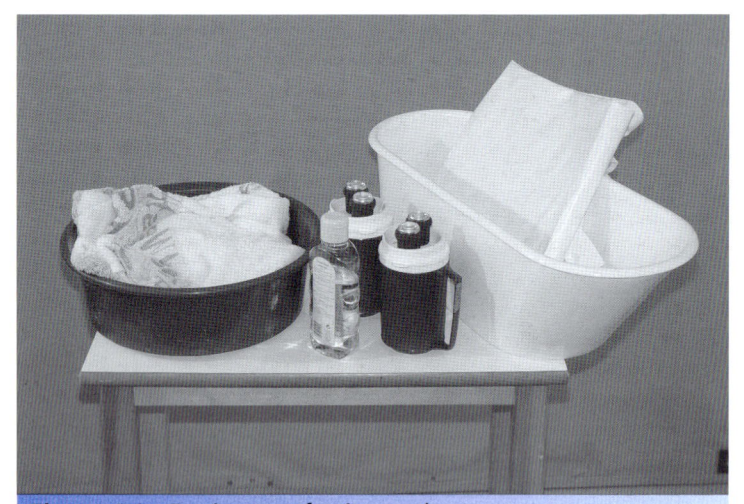

Figure 4.1 Equipment for ice pack.

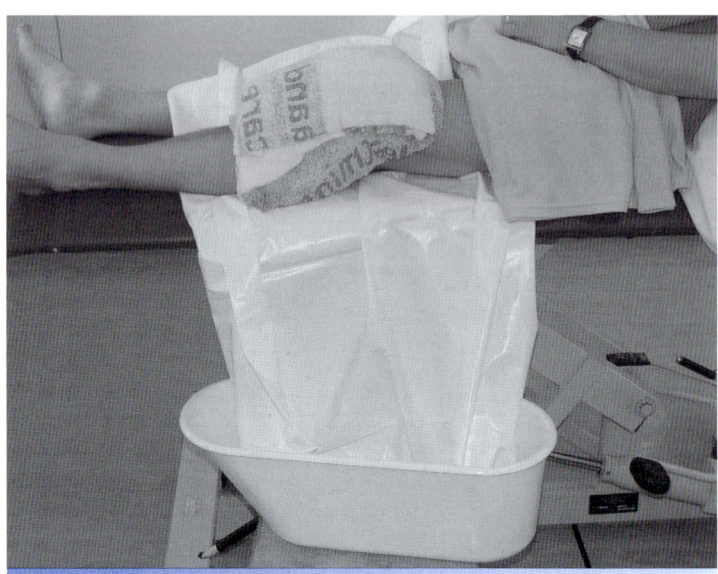

Figure 4.2 Ice pack applied to the knee. Excess water will run into the bath.

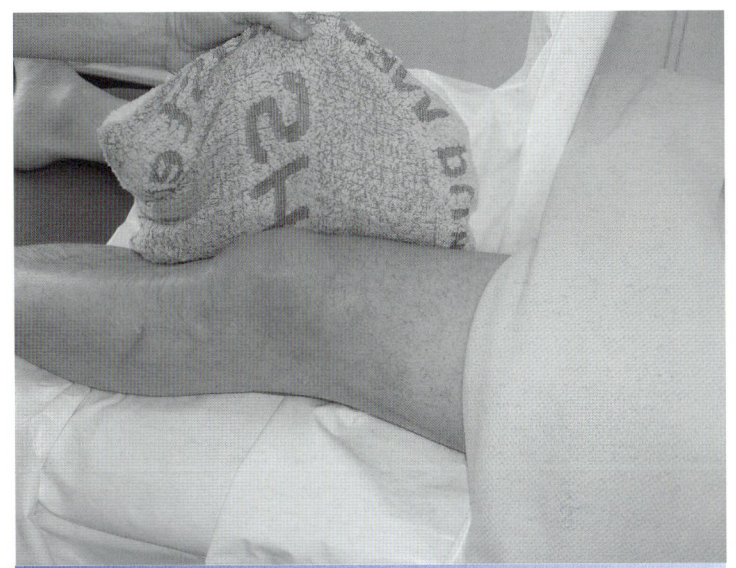

Figure 4.3 The ice pack causes an intense erythema around the knee.

ADAPTATIONS

Ice can also be applied in the ways shown in Figures 4.4 and 4.5.

CRYOCUFF

The cryocuff provides focal compression and cold application to provide optimal control of swelling, and is recommended for use in oedema, haematoma, haemarthrosis and pain.

The reservoir is filled with crushed ice and water. Once the cuff is placed around the limb, it can be connected to the reservoir via an insulated tube. The reservoir should be raised approximately 15 cm above the level of the cuff, which fills with cold water. The water can be circulated with cold by simply lowering the reservoir below the cuff for a short period and then raising again to refill the cuff. Once filled with ice this can be used throughout the day, providing ice is added periodically (see Fig. 4.6).

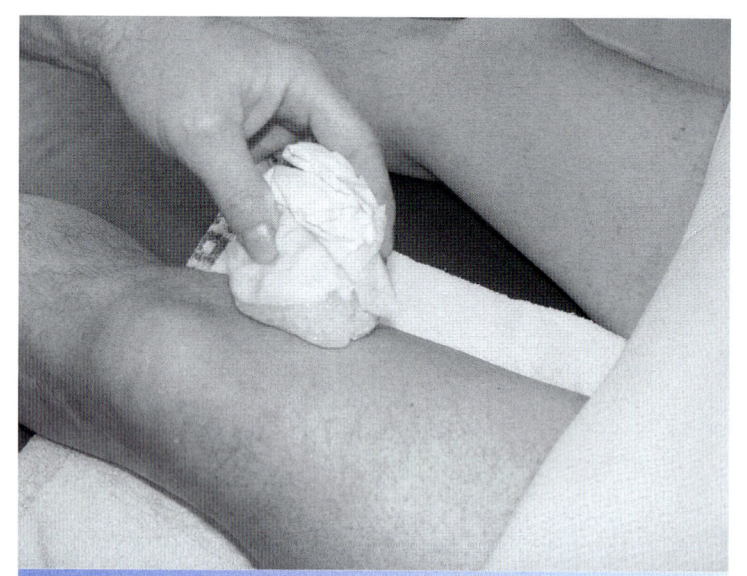

Figure 4.4 Ice massage to medial aspect of the knee. Oil is not required on the skin for this technique. Massage the area in a circular motion for 10 min.

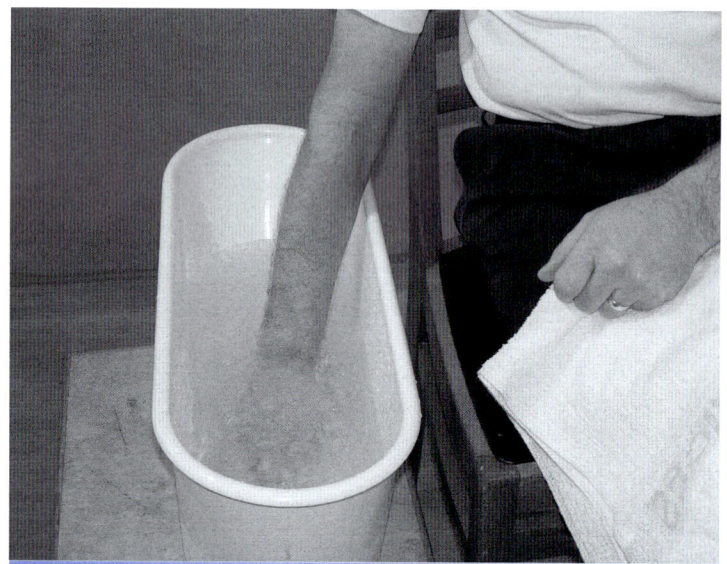

Figure 4.5 Ice immersion using 50% water and 50% crushed ice. Oil is not required. Immersion continues for a total time of 10 min.

Ice/cold packs (cryotherapy) 57

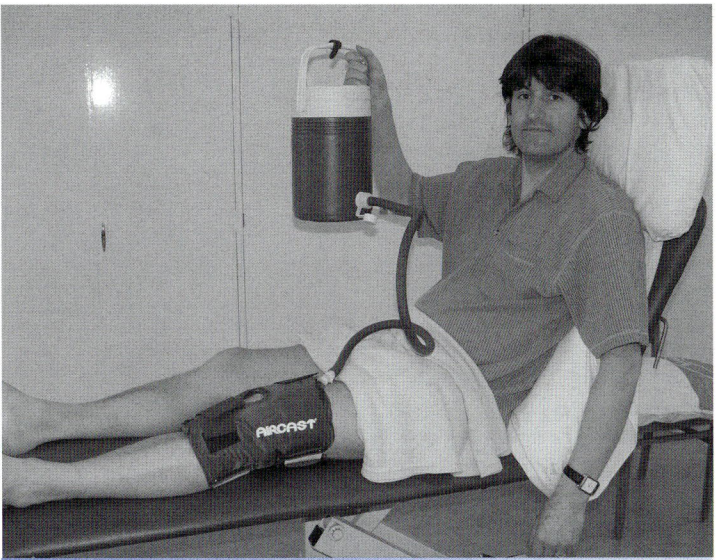

Figure 4.6 Cryocuff to the knee. *Note* the reservoir is held approximately 15 cm above the level of the cuff.

Physiological effects
Vasoconstriction
Decreased blood flow
Increase in blood viscosity
Decreased metabolic rate
Effects on peripheral nerves
Slowed healing.

Therapeutic uses
Decreases oedema production
Reduction of bleeding
Reduces swelling
Minimises inflammation
Reduces muscle spasm/spasticity
Reduces pain
Reduces chronic oedema and joint effusions
Recent injuries and post-surgery.

(See also Robertson et al 2006 and Kitchen 2002.)

Contraindications
Decreased sensation to hot/cold
Arteriosclerosis
Peripheral vascular disease
Cryoglobinaemia
Cold urticaria.

Precautions
Cardiac disease
Defective skin sensation
Skin hypersensitivity
Adverse psychological factors.

(See also Robertson et al 2006 and Kitchen 2002.)

Ice/cold packs (cryotherapy)

Notes

PRACTICAL ELECTROTHERAPY

Treatment record

Table 4.1 *OBSERVATIONAL/REFLECTIVE CHECKLIST*

	Observation	Y/N	Comments
Introduction	Did the therapist introduce him/herself?	☐	☐
	Was an explanation of the procedure given?	☐	☐
	Was the explanation clear and succinct?	☐	☐
	Were the possible dangers highlighted?	☐	☐
	Was consent obtained?	☐	☐
Comfort and safety	Was the patient comfortable?	☐	☐
	Was the therapist's posture compromised?	☐	☐
	Was the position safe for both parties?	☐	☐
	Was the modality applied with due care and attention?	☐	☐
Technique	Were the contraindications checked?	☐	☐
	Were the appropriate tests performed prior to treatment?	☐	☐
	Was an explanation of the physiological effects of the technique offered to the patient?	☐	☐
	Was this explanation accurate?	☐	☐
	Was the technique/modality applied correctly?	☐	☐
	Were the correct times and settings used?	☐	☐
	Was the skin checked after the treatment for adverse effects?	☐	☐

Table 4.2 SUMMARY OF STUDIES INVESTIGATING THE EFFECTIVENESS OF CRYOTHERAPY

Authors	Aim of study	Numbers	Methods	Assessment	Results
Barry et al (2003)	To investigate the current practice after total knee replacement (TKR).	263 responses, routinely applying cryotherapy after TKR.	A questionnaire survey of appropriate physiotherapists in NHS and private hospitals throughout the UK.		Cryotherapy was applied using cryocuff (59%) and crushed ice (30%). Treatment was applied between 24 and 48 h postoperatively, twice daily.
Belitsky et al (1987)	To evaluate the effectiveness of wet ice, dry ice and cryogen packs in reducing skin temperature.	10 healthy females, each received 3 interventions.	1. Wet ice (ice flakes) to calf muscle for 15 min. 2. Dry ice (ice flakes in a plastic bag) to calf for 15 min. 3. Cryogen pack to calf for 15 min.	Skin temperature was measured prior to treatment, immediately after treatment and 15 min after removal of ice pack.	Wet ice (ice flakes) was significantly cooler than both dry ice and cryogen pack, after 15 min of cryotherapy to the calf muscle.
Bleakley et al (2004)	To explore the clinical evidence base for cryotherapy and to investigate five specific objectives.	22 eligible randomised controlled trials were reviewed.	A systematic review of randomised controlled trials was undertaken.		The authors conclude that more high-quality studies are required to ensure that clinicians and sports people are following evidence-based guidelines in the treatment of acute soft-tissue injuries.

Ice/cold packs (cryotherapy)

Authors	Aim of study	Numbers	Methods	Assessment	Results
Buzzard et al (2003)	To compare ice therapy using cryocuff with pulsed shortwave diathermy (PSWD) for the reduction of oedema following calcaneal fractures.	20 patients with acute calcaneal fractures were randomly assigned to receive one of two interventions	Nine patients received PSWD (pulse frequency 26 Hz, pulse duration 200 μs, intensity of 35 W for 15 min) twice daily for 5 days. 11 patients received the ice therapy (cryocuff) for 20 min, 6 times a day for 5 days.	Swelling around the ankle and foot was measured using a tape measure. Range of movement (dorsiflexion, plantarflexion, inversion and aversion) was measured using a goniometer.	All 20 subjects gained a significant increase in all the ankle movements ($p = 0.007$). There was no notable reduction in swelling in either group.
Chartered Society of Physiotherapy (CSP) (1998)	This guideline, produced by the ACPSM, outlines the safest way to use ice/cryotherapy, giving evidence, recommendations and current practice.		Ice should be applied immediately following acute musculoskeletal injury. Chipped/crushed ice in a damp towel is the most effective application. Damp towels should always be applied directly to the skin before using ice packs to avoid an 'ice burn'.	A maximum period of 30 min is recommended. Most effective duration is 20–30 min, applied every 2 h. An athlete should not return to participation immediately following ice. Care should be taken in the application of ice to patients with little subcutaneous fat.	Beware of contraindications to cold therapy: patients with cold-induced hypertension, cold allergy (urticaria, joint pain), Raynaud's syndrome, peripheral vascular disease or sickle cell anaemia.

Authors	Aim of study	Numbers	Methods	Assessment	Results
Chesterton et al (2002)	To compare the cooling effect of a frozen gel pack with frozen peas and a control pack over common clinical treatment times of 10 and 20 min.	20 subjects, each randomly received three interventions.	1. Gel pack to rectus femoris for 20 min. 2. Packet of frozen peas to the same area for 20 min. 3. Control gel pack to the same area for 20 min. These were all placed on a single layer of damp cotton towel to prevent frostbite.	Skin temperature (using a thermistor surface probe) was measured prior to treatment and at 10 min and 20 min after application.	The frozen peas produced significantly greater mean skin temperature reduction after 10 min and 20 min of application.
Cuthill & Cuthill (2006)	This paper describes how an ice burn was sustained after the application of a cold pack. Its aim is to investigate the incidence of cold-induced injury due to the use of ice and to re-assess the cryotherapy practice of physiotherapists in Scotland.	A total of 111 questionnaires were sent to physiotherapists working in private practice throughout Scotland.	The paper describes how a 29-year-old healthy female sustained a soft tissue injury to the gastrocnemius muscle while running. She treated this with a shop-bought cold pack, kept in her home freezer. This was applied with the leg resting on a chair, producing a compressive effect.	The next morning, a large blister appeared over the posterior calf. The patient attended the burns clinic where the burn depth was assessed as a combination of superficial and deep partial thickness. The patient was assessed at the clinic every 48 h and full coverage was completed in 12 days.	80 physiotherapists responded to the questionnaire. All participants advocated the use of ice following soft tissue injuries. Almost all explained how the ice pack should be used. 70/80 used ice immediately after injury, 9/80 within the first 12 h and 1/80 between 12–24 h. 2/77 continued treatment for 24 h,

Ice/cold packs (cryotherapy)

Authors	Aim of study	Numbers	Methods	Assessment	Results
			The pack was kept in position for 30 min. On removing the pack, a large hard and purple patch was noted. This became very painful over the next hour.		25/77 for up to 48 h, 26/77 up to 72 h and 24/77 for longer. 30/78 applied ice for 10 min, 43/78 for 20 min, 4/78 for 30 min and 1/78 for 40 min. All physiotherapists were aware of the possibility of producing an ice-induced burn from cryotherapy.
Dover & Powers (2004)	To assess shoulder joint position sense (JPS) after a 30-min cryotherapy session.	30 healthy subjects were randomly assigned to receive active treatment or control first.	1. Ice pack applied to dominant shoulder for 30 min. 2. Subjects remained in the same position (supine) for 30 min, receiving no ice pack (control).	An inclinometer was used to measure the range of movement (ROM) and JPS testing. JPS was measured before and after receiving either the ice pack or the control (no ice). Skin temperature was measured every 5 min during treatment and immediately after treatment.	No significant differences were found when comparing male and female skin surface temperatures during cryotherapy ($p = 0.100$). Cryotherapy for 30 min to the shoulder does not impair joint position sense (JPS).

Authors	Aim of study	Numbers	Methods	Assessment	Results
Graham & Stevenson (2000)	This is a case report of a female physical education teacher presenting to the A&E department with a frostbite injury to the dorsum of her left foot. The patient had a 4-week history of discomfort to her left foot. She applied a bag of frozen chips, wrapped in a towel, to the dorsum of her foot in an attempt to relieve the discomfort. She then fell asleep and left the frozen chips in contact with her foot for 40 min. On awakening, the discomfort had resolved but there was a noticeable erythema where the frozen chips had been applied. She sought help from her GP and was subsequently sent to A&E. Full recovery ensued after surgical excision of the necrotic tissue and split skin grafting. Patients must be reminded of the dangers of cryotherapy as well as the benefits.				
Hubbard et al (2004)	To search the literature for papers on the effect of cryotherapy on return to participation after injury.	Four studies were identified and reviewed by the authors.	The authors performed an extensive search of the literature from 1976 to 2003 for literature related to cryotherapy application. Key words were: cryotherapy, return to participation, cold treatment, ice injury, sport, oedema and pain.	The Physiotherapy Evidence Database (PEDro) scale was used to rate the papers.	The authors concluded that cryotherapy had a positive effect on return to participation but further research was necessary before the effect of cryotherapy on return to participation could be fully elucidated.

Authors	Aim of study	Numbers	Methods	Assessment	Results
Janwantanakul (2004)	To investigate the different rate of cooling time and magnitude of cooling temperature during ice bag treatment with and without damp towel wrap.	30 healthy females, each received three interventions.	1. Chipped ice in a plastic bag, to the rectus femoris for 20 min. 2. Chipped ice in a plastic bag and wrapped in a single layer of damp towelling, to same area for 20 min. 3. Plastic bag containing water at room temperature, applied to same area for 20 min.	Skin surface temperature was measured every minute for the 20 min of application.	The ice bag applied directly to the skin led to a greater surface temperature reduction.
Kauranen & Vanharanta (1997)	To evaluate the effects of hot and cold packs on motor performance of normal hands.	20 healthy female students.	All subjects received a hot pack for 20 min to forearm and hand. They later received a cold pack for 15 min to the same area.	Four hand tests (reaction time, movement speed, tapping time and coordination), taken immediately, 15 min and 30 min after treatment.	Hot pack treatment delayed simple reaction time and increased tapping speed. Cold treatment delayed simple reaction time, speed of movement and tapping time.

Authors	Aim of study	Numbers	Methods	Assessment	Results
MacAuley (2001)	To examine various treatment protocols and to identify the specific advice on duration, frequency and mode of application of ice in acute soft tissue injury across a range of textbooks.	45 textbooks were included in the study.	A systematic research of a sample of textbooks was undertaken by the author. The search was designed to identify specific aspects of ice therapy; duration, frequency and mode of application.		In 17 of the textbooks, there was no specific guidance on the duration, frequency or length of ice treatment. Advice on treatment duration was given in 28 texts, and in many of these the recommendations differed depending on the particular ice therapy, injury location, or severity. Similarly, advice on the frequency of treatment was available in 21 texts, and 22 advised on the optimum length of treatment.
Malone et al (1992)	To present six case studies of cryotherapy-induced peripheral nerve injuries in athletes.		The case studies involved three peroneal nerve injuries, two lateral cutaneous nerve of thigh injuries and one supraclavicular nerve injury. The duration of ice treatment was from 15–60 min. The duration of disability ranged from 1 h to 6 months. All the patients gained full recovery. The authors do comment that these		

Ice/cold packs (cryotherapy)

Authors	Aim of study	Numbers	Methods	Assessment	Results
Martin et al (2001)	To prospectively evaluate the intra-articular temperature of the knee to see whether a significant decline occurs with postoperative application of cryotherapy after routine arthroscopy.	17 patients undergoing arthroscopic surgery were placed in either a treatment group or the control group.	*The Treatment Group:* (12 subjects) immediately postoperatively, received cryotherapy to the knee (cryocuff) continuously for 2 h. Ice water was exchanged in the cuff every 30 min. *The Control Group:* (5 subjects) were fitted with the cryocuff, which was kept empty for the first hour and filled with ice water for the second hour.	Thigh circumference was measured in each patient 10 cm above the superior pole of the patella. A thermocouple probe was placed intra-articularly, into the lateral gutter of the knee and the temperature was recorded every minute for 2 h.	The temperature in the treatment group declined significantly over the 2 h ($p = 0.008$). The temperature in the control group significantly increased over the first hour ($p = 0.006$) and significantly decreased after the ice was applied ($p = 0.06$).
Morsi (2002)	To investigate the effect of cryotherapy after total knee arthroplasty (TKA) on range of movement, haemovac drainage and blood loss, VAS pain score, analgesic consumption and wound healing.	30 patients undergoing bilateral TKAs, each receiving two interventions.	1. Continuous flow cold therapy, continuously for 6 days. 2. TKA to the opposite limb did not receive cold therapy.	Visual analogue scale (VAS), analgesic consumption, haemovac output and blood loss, range of movement and wound healing.	The cold therapy provided greater knee extension and flexion at 1 week postoperatively. It also resulted in a lower volume of haemovac output and blood loss, lower VAS pain score, analgesic consumption, with no adverse effect on wound healing.

Authors	Aim of study	Numbers	Methods	Assessment	Results
O'Toole & Rayatt (1999)	This is a case report of a 59-year-old woman presenting to the A&E department with a superficial partial thickness burn to her calf. The woman strained her calf muscle while using a treadmill at the gym. A member of staff advised her to put an ice pack directly onto the calf instead of telling her to put some material in between. The woman rested her leg for 20 min with the ice pack underneath her calf. The next day a huge blister developed on her calf and after 4 days, she went to A&E. She was treated at the Burns and Plastics Unit and healed after 10 days. The authors conclude that awareness of the risk of this type of injury is important for all those entrusted with advising patients on the treatment of minor soft tissue injuries.				
Steen et al (2000)	To compare the effectiveness of ice pack and Epifoam with cooling maternity gel pads at alleviating postnatal perineal trauma.	120 patients with perineal trauma were randomly allocated to one of three interventions.	1. Ice packs (38 subjects). 2. Epifoam (42 subjects). 3. Gel pads (40 subjects).	Measurement outcomes were: levels of oedema, bruising and self-assessed pain.	The gel pads were more effective in alleviating perineal trauma when compared with the other regimens and were more highly rated by women.

Authors	Aim of study	Numbers	Methods	Assessment	Results
Uchio et al (2003)	To investigate whether cryotherapy influences laxity, stiffness and joint position sense (JPS) of the knee joint.	20 healthy volunteers.	All participants had a cooling pad applied to one knee for 15 min (temperature maintained at 4°C). The cooling pad was applied to the other knee 2 days later.	Anteroposterior (AP) knee laxity and anterior terminal stiffness (ATS) were measured by a knee arthrometer at pre-test, immediately after the cooling intervention and 15 min later. Joint position sense was measured using a Cybex dynamometer before and after cooling.	The AP knee laxity declined significantly after 15 min of cooling. ATS increased significantly after cooling. At 15 min of cooling of the knee joint, the ability to accurately reproduce the target angle decreased.
Waters & Raisler (2003)	To investigate the use of ice massage for reduction of labour pain.	49 patients, all at the early stage of labour.	Ice massage was given to the hand (LI 4) for 20 min or throughout 3–4 contractions. It was then repeated on the other hand.	Visual analogue scale (VAS) measured pain intensity before the ice intervention and during ice intervention. The participants also scored a McGill Pain Questionnaire (MPQ) within 24 h after the delivery.	Ice massage produced a mean pain reduction on the VAS of 28.22 mm on the left hand and 11.93 mm on the right hand. The MPQ score reduced from 3 (distressing) to 2 (discomfort).

REFERENCES

Barry B, Wallace L, Lamb S 2003 Cryotherapy after total knee replacement: a survey of current practice. Physiotherapy Research International 8:111–120

Belitsky R B, Odam S J, Huble-Kozey C 1987 Evaluation of the effectiveness of wet ice, dry ice, and cryogen packs in reducing skin temperature. Physical Therapy 67:1080–1084

Bleakley C, McDonough S, MacAuley D 2004 The use of ice in the treatment of acute soft-tissue injury: A systematic review of randomized controlled trials. American Journal of Sports Medicine 32:251–261

Buzzard B M, Pratt R K, Briggs P J et al 2003 Is pulsed short wave diathermy better than ice therapy for the reduction of oedema following calcaneal fractures? Physiotherapy 89:734–742

Chartered Society of Physiotherapy (CSP) 1998 Guideline 3 – Ice. Association of Chartered Physiotherapists in Sports Medicine. CSP, London. Online. Available: www.csp.org.uk

Chesterton L S, Foster N E, Ross L 2002 Skin temperature response to cryotherapy. Archives of Physical Medicine and Rehabilitation 83:543–549

Cuthill J A, Cuthill G S 2006 Partial-thickness burn to the leg following application of a cold pack: case report and result of a questionnaire survey of Scottish physiotherapists in private practice. Physiotherapy 92:61–65

Dover G, Powers M E 2004 Cryotherapy does not impair shoulder joint position sense. Archives of Physical Medicine and Rehabilitation 85:1241–1246

Graham C A, Stevenson J 2000 Frozen chips: an unusual cause of severe frostbite injury. British Journal of Sports Medicine 34:382–384

Hubbard T J, Aronson S L, Denegar C R 2004 Does cryotherapy hasten return to participation? A systematic review. Journal of Athletic Training 39:88–94

Janwantanakul P 2004 Different rate of cooling time and magnitude of cooling temperature during ice bag treatment with and without damp towel wrap. Physical Therapy in Sport 5:156–161

Kauranen K, Vanharanta H 1997 Effects of hot and cold packs on motor performance of normal hands. Physiotherapy 83:340–344

Kitchen S 2002 Heat and cold: conduction methods. In: Kitchen S (ed) Electrotherapy: evidence-based practice, 11th edn. Churchill Livingstone, London, p 129–136

MacAuley D 2001 Do textbooks agree on their advice on ice? Clinical Journal of Sport Medicine 11:67–72

Malone T R, Engelhardt D L, Kirkpatrick J S et al 1992 Nerve injury in athletes caused by cryotherapy. Journal of Athletic Training 27:235–237

Martin S S, Spindler K P, Tarter J W et al 2001 Cryotherapy: an effective modality for decreasing intra-articular temperature after knee arthroscopy. American Journal of Sports Medicine 29:288–291

Morsi E 2002 Continuous-flow cold therapy after total knee arthroplasty. Journal of Arthroplasty 17:718–722

O'Toole G, Rayatt S 1999 Frostbite at the gym: a case report of an ice pack burn. British Journal of Sports Medicine 33:278–279

Robertson V, Ward A, Low J et al 2006 Electrotherapy explained: principles and practice, 4th edn. Elsevier Science, Oxford

Steen M, Cooper K, Marchant P et al 2000 A randomised controlled trial to compare the effectiveness of icepack and Epifoam with cooling maternity gel pads at alleviating postnatal perineal trauma. Midwifery 16:48–55

Uchio Y, Ochi M, Fujihara A et al 2003 Cryotherapy influences joint laxity and position sense of the healthy knee joint. Archives of Physical Medicine and Rehabilitation 84:131–135

Waters B L, Raisler J 2003 Ice massage for reduction of labor pain. Journal of Midwifery & Women's Health 48:317–321

PART 2

ELECTRICAL STIMULATION

Chapter 5 – Transcutaneous electrical nerve stimulation   77

Chapter 6 – Neuromuscular electrical stimulation   103

Chapter 7 – Interferential therapy   137

CHAPTER 5

Transcutaneous electrical nerve stimulation

PRODUCTION

Transcutaneous electrical nerve stimulation (TENS) is a simple battery powered device, which transmits a low frequency electrical impulse and is applied to the skin via lead wires and surface electrodes (Robertson et al 2006, Johnson 2002).

EQUIPMENT

TENS machine
Battery
Self-adhesive electrodes (2 or 4)
Leads
Neurotips for pin-prick (sharp/blunt) testing.

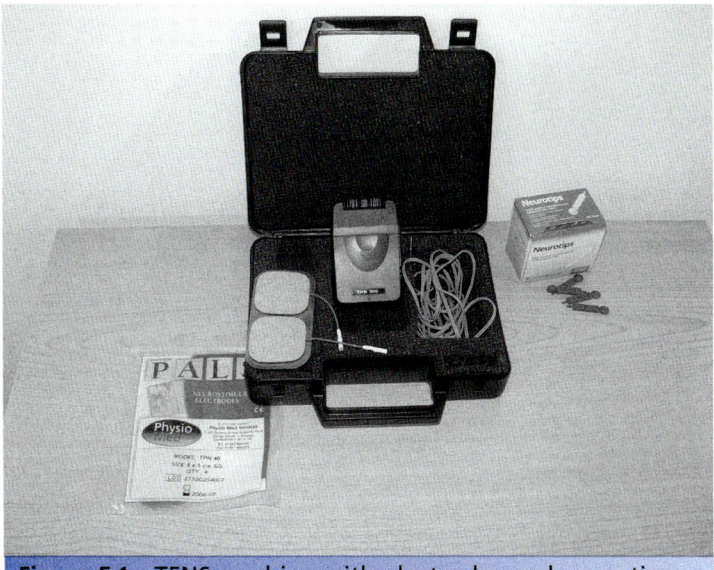

Figure 5.1 TENS machine with electrodes and neurotips.

PRACTICAL ELECTROTHERAPY

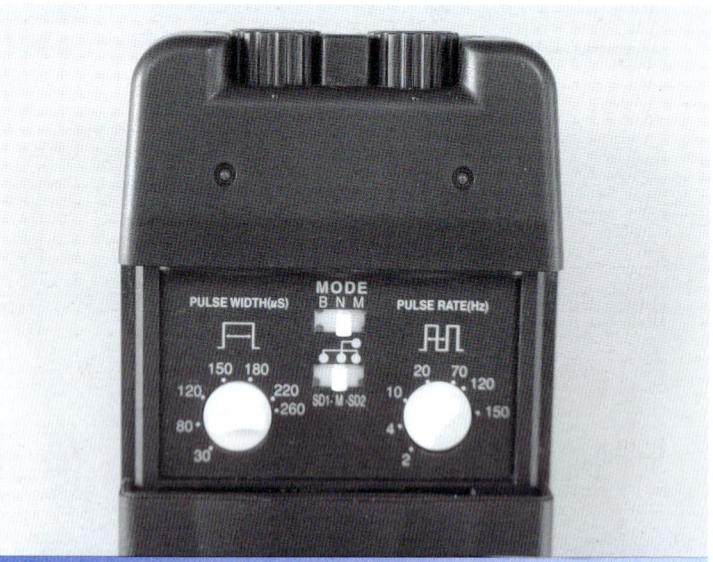

Figure 5.2 TENS machine showing dials to alter the settings. The left-hand dial indicates the pulse width (30–250 μs). The right-hand dial indicates the pulse rate/frequency (2–150 Hz). Mode: N, normal; B, burst; M, modulated.

SETTINGS
Conventional (High) TENS
Frequency (pulse rate): 150 Hz
Pulse width: 50–80 μs, 8 h+
Tingling/pins and needles sensation felt.

Acupuncture (Low) TENS
Frequency (pulse rate): 1–4 Hz
Pulse width: 200 μs, 30 min
Sharp, pricking sensation (very strong) felt, plus muscle twitch seen.

APPLICATION OF TENS TO THE CERVICAL SPINE
1. Expose the area of application and ensure that it is clean.
2. Explain the procedure and gain informed consent.
3. Check for any contraindications.
4. Perform a pin-prick test.

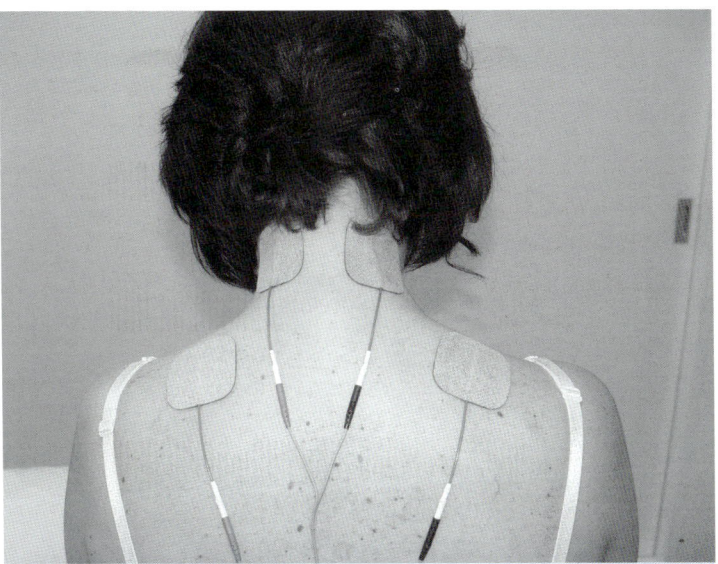

Figure 5.3 Electrode placement for neck pain. Electrodes placed over the cervical nerve roots and GB 21, an acupuncture point.

5. Place electrode either side of the area to be treated (Fig. 5.3).
6. Attach the leads to the machine.
7. Set the desired frequency and pulse rate.
8. Turn up the intensity as much as the patient can tolerate comfortably.
9. Start the timer.
10. At the end of the time, turn the machine off and remove the electrodes, checking the skin for any signs of adverse reactions.
11. The patient may have to be taught how to apply and use the machine, as TENS is frequently given for home use.

ADAPTATIONS

TENS can be used with two or four electrodes, depending on the size of the area to be treated.

ELECTRODE PLACEMENTS
Close to where the pain is perceived
At appropriate acupuncture or trigger points (see Fig. 5.4)
Over the spinal nerve roots, close to the spinous process
Within the same dermatome, myotome or sclerotome.

Physiological effects
Both modes of stimulation are used to produce pain relief.

- High TENS stimulates the Aβ fibres and analgesia is produced by the pain gate theory.
- Low TENS stimulates Aδ and C fibres which produces pain relief via the descending inhibitory pathway (Robertson et al 2006).

Contraindications
Treatment over or close to a pacemaker
Heart disease or arrhythmias
Undiagnosed pain
Epilepsy
Infections
Deep X-ray therapy
Tumours.

Do not apply the electrodes to the following areas:
Mouth
Carotid sinus
Broken skin
Anaesthetised skin
The abdomen during pregnancy
Near the eyes.

(See Robertson et al 2006, Johnson 2002.)

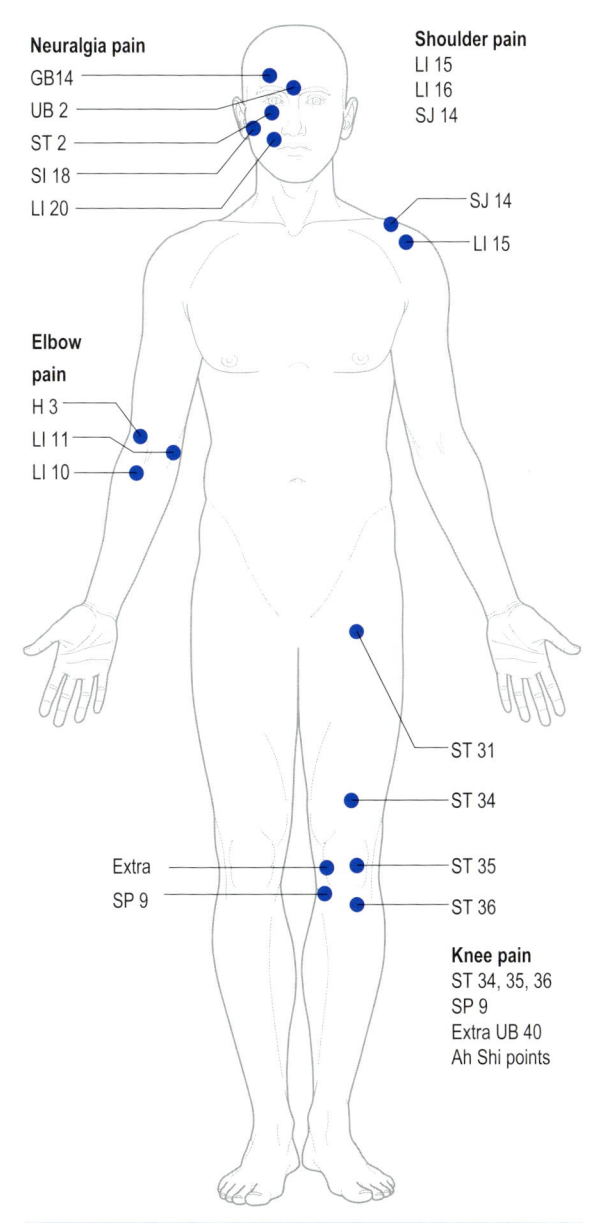

Transcutaneous electrical nerve stimulation 81

Neuralgia pain
GB14
UB 2
ST 2
SI 18
LI 20

Shoulder pain
LI 15
LI 16
SJ 14

SJ 14
LI 15

Elbow pain
H 3
LI 11
LI 10

ST 31
ST 34
Extra — ST 35
SP 9 — ST 36

Knee pain
ST 34, 35, 36
SP 9
Extra UB 40
Ah Shi points

Figure 5.4 Body charts outlining the acupuncture points used with TENS.

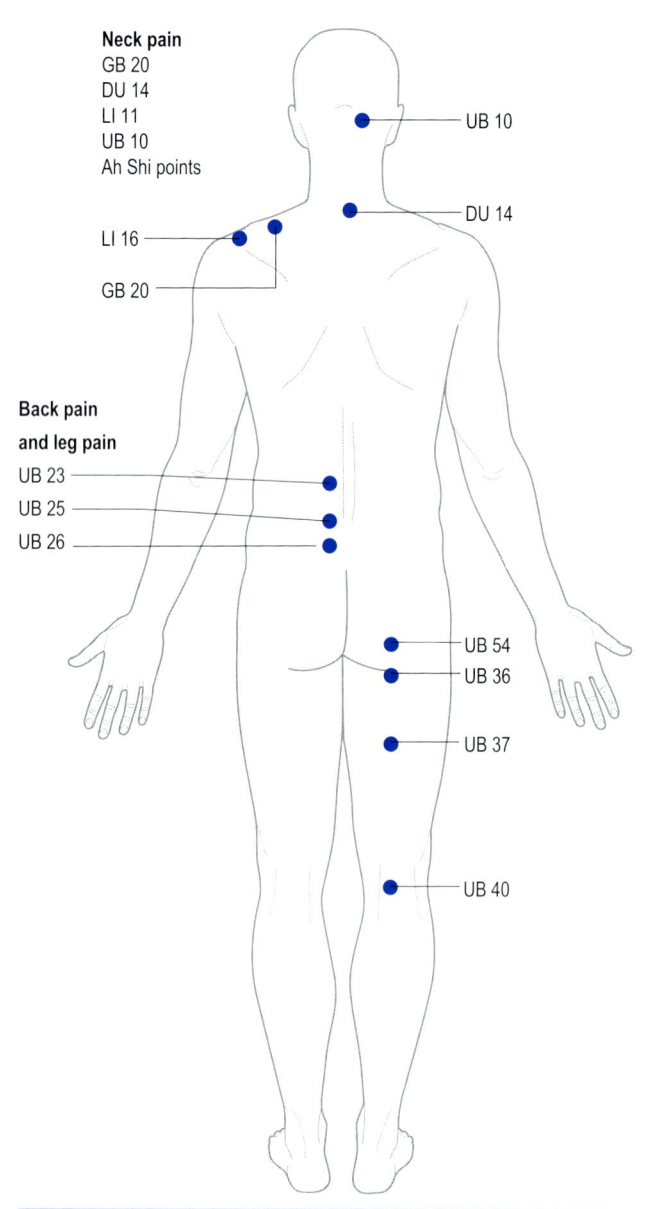

Figure 5.4, cont'd

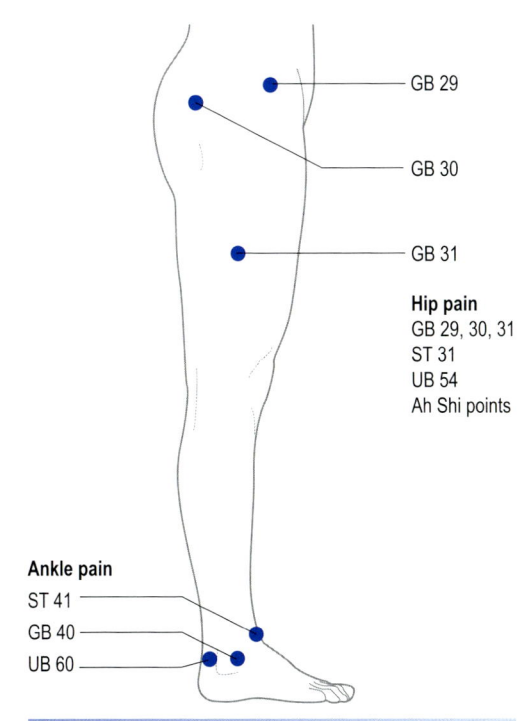

Transcutaneous electrical nerve stimulation 83

- GB 29
- GB 30
- GB 31

Hip pain
GB 29, 30, 31
ST 31
UB 54
Ah Shi points

Ankle pain
ST 41
GB 40
UB 60

Figure 5.4, cont'd

Notes

Transcutaneous electrical nerve stimulation

Treatment record

PRACTICAL ELECTROTHERAPY

Table 5.1 *OBSERVATIONAL/REFLECTIVE CHECKLIST*

	Observation	Y/N	Comments
Introduction	Did the therapist introduce him/herself?	☐	☐
	Was an explanation of the procedure given?	☐	☐
	Was the explanation clear and succinct?	☐	☐
	Were the possible dangers highlighted?	☐	☐
	Was consent obtained?	☐	☐
Comfort and safety	Was the patient comfortable?	☐	☐
	Was the therapist's posture compromised?	☐	☐
	Was the position safe for both parties?	☐	☐
	Was the modality applied with due care and attention?	☐	☐
Technique	Were the contraindications checked?	☐	☐
	Were the appropriate tests performed prior to treatment?	☐	☐
	Was an explanation of the physiological effects of the technique offered to the patient?	☐	☐
	Was this explanation accurate?	☐	☐
	Was the technique/modality applied correctly?	☐	☐
	Were the correct times and settings used?	☐	☐
	Was the skin checked after the treatment for adverse effects?	☐	☐

Authors	Aim of study	Numbers	Methods	Assessment	Results
Anderson et al (2004)	To assess whether chronic low frequency electrical stimulation (CLFES) to the calf muscles of patients with intermittent claudication could improve walking ability and muscle function.	30 patients with stable claudication were divided into two groups.	15 patients received active CLFES (square wave pulses, 250 μs duration, 100 V, and frequency 6 Hz to produce a visible muscle contraction) to the calf muscles for 20 min, three times a day for 4 weeks. 15 patients (control) received TENS (50 μs, 100 V and frequency of 90 Hz) to produce a tingling sensation without a muscle contraction to the calf muscle for 20 min, three times a day for 4 weeks.	All the subjects were assessed by treadmill to determine claudication and maximal walking distances, and resting and post-exercise ankle–brachial pressure index (ABPI). Calf muscle function was tested during 5 min of electrically evoked twitch contractions, where strain gauges were used to measure isometric plantarflexion torque.	There were significant improvements in treadmill performance for those patients who had received CLFES. There was a significant increase in pain-free walking distance ($p < 0.001$) and maximum walking distance ($p < 0.05$) while the control treatment showed no effect.
Breit & van der Wall (2004)	To evaluate the effects of TENS for postoperative relief of pain after total knee arthroplasty (TKA).	69 patients undergoing TKA were randomly allocated to three groups.	*Group 1:* (22 patients) received patient-controlled analgesia (PCA) only for postoperative pain relief. *Group 2:* (25 patients) received PCA and TENS (set to a maximum output level and *in situ* for 24 h) for postoperative pain relief. *Group 3:* (22 patients) received PCA and sham TENS for postoperative pain relief.	The outcome measure used was the total postoperative morphine dose used over the 24 h period for each of the groups. (Data collected from VAS proved unreliable.)	There was no significant reduction in the requirement for PCA with or without TENS. No TENS parameters were given. There was no indication of how morphine was controlled.

Authors	Aim of study	Numbers	Methods	Assessment	Results
Brosseau et al (2002)	To evaluate the efficacy of different types of TENS compared with placebo on pain relief and other outcome measures for treating patients with rheumatoid arthritis (RA).	Three studies were reviewed by the authors.	The authors undertook a systematic search of the literature. The three studies were RCTs and were reviewed by the authors.		The reviewers conclude that both conventional and acupuncture-like TENS have either statistically or clinically significant benefit over placebo for RA disability.
Brosseau et al (2004)	To evaluate the effectiveness of TENS in the treatment of osteoarthritis (OA) of the lower extremities.	Six studies were reviewed by the authors.	The authors undertook a systematic search of the literature. Six studies were randomised controlled trials (RCTs) and were reviewed by the authors.	The authors outline five basic methods of administrating TENS. (1) Conventional TENS, high frequency (150 Hz), short pulse duration (<50 μs), low intensity, administered periodically throughout the day, usually for 30 min periods. (2) Acupuncture-like TENS (AL-TENS), low frequency (1–10 Hz), long pulse duration (>150 μs), and a high intensity, close to the patients' limit of tolerance.	All modes of TENS showed a significant benefit for pain relief in the treatment of OA involving the knee and/or hip.

Authors	Aim of study	Numbers	Methods	Assessment	Results
				(3) Burst TENS (BTENS), which is characterised by low-frequency (<10 Hz) burst impulses at low intensity. (4) Brief-intense TENS (BITENS): pulses of long duration (>150 µs) given at high frequency (>80 Hz). (5) Modulation TENS, where all characteristics of the stimulus are variable.	
Carroll et al (1997)	To evaluate the effectiveness and safety of transcutaneous electrical nerve stimulation (TENS) in labour: a systematic review.	Eight studies were reviewed by the authors.	The authors undertook a systematic search of the literature. Eight studies were RCTs and were reviewed by the authors.		The authors conclude that there is no compelling evidence for TENS having any analgesic effect during labour.

Authors	Aim of study	Numbers	Methods	Assessment	Results
Cheing et al (2002)	To evaluate the cumulative effect of repeated TENS on chronic OA of the knee pain over a 4-week treatment period, comparing it with that of placebo stimulation and exercise training given alone or in combination with TENS.	66 patients with OA of the knee were randomly assigned to four groups.	*Group 1:* (16 subjects) received conventional TENS (frequency of 80 Hz, pulse width 140 µs, daily for 60 min. *Group 2:* (16 subjects) received sham TENS for the same duration. *Group 3:* (15 subjects) received isometric exercise training for 20 min. *Group 4:* (15 subjects) received active TENS and isometric muscle training. All subjects received treatment 5 days a week for 4 weeks (20 sessions).	The visual analogue scale (VAS) was used to measure knee pain intensity before and after each treatment session over a 4-week period, and at the 4-week follow-up session.	The four treatment protocols did not show significant between-group differences over the study period.

Authors	Aim of study	Numbers	Methods	Assessment	Results
Chesterton et al (2003)	To determine the effects of a comprehensive range of parameter combinations (frequency, intensity and stimulation site) on an experimental model of pressure pain threshold (PPT) on healthy volunteers.	180 subjects were randomised into six active TENS groups. Control and sham data (60) were utilised from a previous study.	Two TENS frequencies (4 Hz or 110 Hz) and two intensities (strong but comfortable or highest tolerable) at a fixed pulse duration (200 μs) were applied at three sites relative to the measurement site (segmentally, extrasegmentally or a combination of these), for 30 min.	Pain pressure threshold (PPT) to the first dorsal interosseous muscle was measured, using an algometer, before TENS application and at 10 min intervals over a 60 min period.	The high frequency, high intensity segmental and combined stimulation groups showed rapid onset and significant hypoalgesic effects.
Chiu et al (2005)	To investigate the effects of TENS on acupuncture points and a neck exercise programme in patients with chronic neck pain.	218 patients with chronic neck pain were randomly allocated to three groups.	*Group 1:* (78 subjects) received infrared radiation (IRR) for 20 min and advice on neck care, twice weekly for 6 weeks. *Group 2:* (73 subjects) received IRR for 20 min and neck care advice, plus TENS (4 electrodes, frequency of 80 Hz, pulse duration 150 μs, producing a tingling sensation) for 30 min. *Group 3:* (67 subjects) received IRR for 20 min	Patients were assessed by the verbal numerical pain scale for pain; the Northwick Park Neck Pain Questionnaire for neck disability scores; and the peak isometric strength of the neck muscles. Secondary outcome included percentage of subjects taking medication and sick leave because of the neck pain. Patients were assessed pre-treatment, post-treatment and at 6 months follow-up.	The results demonstrated that after treatment, significant improvement in the verbal numerical pain scale was found in the TENS group ($p = 0.027$) and exercise group ($p < 0.001$). A significant reduction in the Northwick Park

Authors	Aim of study	Numbers	Methods	Assessment	Results
			and neck care advice plus an intensive neck exercise programme for 35 min. All participants attended twice weekly for 6 weeks.		Neck Pain Questionnaire was found in all three groups. A significant improvement was also found in neck muscle strength in all three groups. All the improvements in the intervention groups were maintained at the 6-month follow-up.
Johnson (1998)	This is an extensive review, discussing the analgesic effects and clinical effectiveness of acupuncture-like TENS (AL-TENS).				
Kaplan et al (1998)	To examine the effectiveness of TENS for pain relief during labour and delivery.	104 patients received a TENS device during labour.	All participants received a TENS device, fitted with obstetric electrodes (lateral to midline between T10 and S2).	The participants completed a questionnaire to evaluate TENS efficacy in relieving pain during labour and delivery (VAS: 1–10).	The majority of patients found TENS effective during the first stage of labour.
Kaye & Brandstater (2005)	This paper discusses pain mechanisms produced by TENS, the settings used clinically, and three methods of administrating TENS (conventional TENS, acupuncture-like TENS and burst TENS). The indications for the use of TENS and its contraindications are also reported.				

Authors	Aim of study	Numbers	Methods	Assessment	Results
Khadilkar et al (2005)	The aim of this systematic review was to determine the effectiveness of TENS in the management of chronic low back pain.		The authors undertook a systematic search of the literature. Two studies were RCTs and were reviewed by the authors.		The authors conclude that the evidence is inconsistent regarding the effectiveness of TENS in reducing pain and improving functional status in patients with chronic LBP.
Köke et al (2004)	To compare the pain reducing effects of three types of TENS in patients with chronic pain.	180 patients with chronic pain were randomly assigned to three groups.	*Group 1:* (29 subjects) received high frequency, low intensity TENS (frequency 80 Hz, pulse duration 80 μs) 4–6 times a day for 1 h periods at sensory threshold intensity. *Group 2:* (30 subjects) received high frequency, high intensity TENS (frequency 80 Hz, pulse duration 250 μs) 4–6 times a day for 30 min periods at maximum tolerable intensity.	Outcome measures used were the patients' global assessment of overall result (the patients' decision to carry on treatment) and the visual analogue scale (VAS) for pain.	No differences in positive assessment of TENS by chronic pain patients or hypoalgesic effects were found between the three different types of TENS.

Authors	Aim of study	Numbers	Methods	Assessment	Results
			Group 3: (121 subjects) received control TENS (frequency 30 Hz, pulse duration 250 μs) choosing duration and intensity as they preferred.		
Miller et al (2005)			This paper reviews the results of studies undertaken to date, evaluating not only the effects of TENS on spasticity, but also the impact of different TENS parameters on its overall effectiveness.		The authors conclude that the results from studies evaluating the effects of TENS on spasticity are favourable. They also suggest that TENS may be particularly helpful for those patients suffering from muscle spasm.

Authors	Aim of study	Numbers	Methods	Assessment	Results
Moore and Shurman (1997)	To evaluate the use of neuromuscular electrical stimulation (NMES) and combining NMES and TENS for the management of chronic back pain.	24 patients with chronic back pain each received four different interventions randomly allocated.	1. TENS (frequency 100 Hz, pulse width 100 µs, amplitude producing a comfortable tingling sensation) to the low back for 5 consecutive hours/day for 2 consecutive days. 2. NMES (frequency 70 Hz, pulse width 200 µs, on/off – 5/15 s, amplitude producing a strong and perceptible contraction of the muscles) to the back. They received three 10-min periods of stimulation over a 5-h period, for 2 consecutive days. 3. Combined TENS/NMES (same parameters as above) to the back. They received, alternatively, one	Each participant completed the Present Pain Intensity (PPI) portion of the McGill Pain Questionnaire and a visual analogue scale (VAS) before and after each treatment.	Combined treatment, TENS and NMES each produced significant pre-treatment to post-treatment reductions in PPI and VAS scores. Combined treatment was superior to both TENS and NMES for pain reduction and pain relief. The authors conclude that a regimen of TENS and NMES may be a valuable adjunct in the management of chronic back pain.

Authors	Aim of study	Numbers	Methods	Assessment	Results
			10-min and one 20-min period of NMES with three periods of TENS stimulation over a 5-h period, for 2 consecutive days. 4. Placebo TENS for 5 h/day for 2 consecutive days. There was a 2-day hiatus period between each intervention to minimise carry-over effects.		
Ng et al (2003)	To evaluate the effect of electro-acupuncture (EA) and TENS in the treatment of osteoarthritis (OA) of the knee in a group of older adults.	24 patients with OA knee pain were randomised into three groups.	*Group 1:* (8 subjects) received EA to acupuncture points ST 35 and EX-LE 4 for 20 min. *Group 2:* (8 subjects) received TENS (frequency 2 Hz, pulse duration 200 μs at a strong sensation, producing a visible muscle contraction) for 20 min.	Subjects were assessed on three occasions: prior to first session, after eight treatments and 2 weeks after the last treatment. Each participant was assessed for pain (numerical rating scale), passive range of knee movement and the Timed-Up-and-Go-Test (TUGT).	There was a significant reduction in knee pain in both EA and TENS groups.

Authors	Aim of study	Numbers	Methods	Assessment	Results
			Group 3: (8 subjects) received education on OA knee care. Treatment was carried out on alternate days for 8 sessions within 2 weeks.		
Sluka & Walsh (2003)	This review describes the basic science mechanisms in support of the different frequencies of TENS stimulation		This paper explains how TENS is used clinically, its effect on pain through the gate control theory of pain and through the descending inhibitory pathways, stimulating the release of endogenous opioids. The authors discuss the literature which supports and refutes each of these theories of pain control. They also discuss the clinical effectiveness of		The authors conclude by saying that the effectiveness of TENS will remain questionable until there is sufficient numbers of high quality, randomised, controlled clinical trials published.

Authors	Aim of study	Numbers	Methods	Assessment	Results
			TENS, reviewing the literature for the use of TENS for chronic pain, chronic low back pain, post-stroke shoulder pain, primary dysmenorrhoea, knee osteoarthritis, acute postoperative pain and labour pain.		
Walsh (1996)	This review discusses four TENS modes used in clinical practice: conventional TENS, acupuncture-like TENS, burst train TENS and brief, intense TENS. It also outlines the common electrode placement sites and in particular focuses on studies which have applied transcutaneous electrical nerve stimulation (TENS) over acupuncture points for a range of conditions.				

Authors	Aim of study	Numbers	Methods	Assessment	Results
Wilson et al (2002)	The aim of this review was to determine whether transcutaneous electrical nerve stimulation (TENS) is an effective treatment for pain relief in people with low back pain.	11 studies were reviewed by the authors.	The authors undertook a systematic search of the literature. A total of 11 studies, RCTs and clinical trials were reviewed by the authors.		Only one of the studies found that TENS was ineffective for reduction of pain. There was a general consensus to support the use of TENS in low back pain. The authors conclude that there is a need to study the effects of different TENS parameters (time, pulse duration, intensity and frequency) on the different types of low back pain.

Authors	Aim of study	Numbers	Methods	Assessment	Results
Yozbatiran et al (2006)	To investigate the effects of short-term electrical stimulation (TENS) in conjunction with neurodevelopment exercises, on sensorimotor and functional recovery of hemiparetic upper limb in acute stroke patients.	36 acute stroke patients were alternately assigned to one of two groups.	*Group 1:* (18 subjects) received 1 h of physical therapy/day and TENS (frequency of 2 Hz, pulse width 260 µs and at an intensity set at the minimum level required to produce full wrist and finger extension for 1 h/day) for a total of 10 days. *Group 2:* (18 subjects) received 1 h of physical therapy/day for 10 days.	Each patient was assessed initially and at discharge using kinaesthesia sense and position sense tests, hand function and hand movement tests.	The results of the study indicated that additional stimulation of the hand and fingers leads to an improved sensorimotor outcome immediately after the intervention.

REFERENCES

Anderson S I, Whatling P, Hudlicka O et al 2004 Chronic transcutaneous electrical stimulation of calf muscles improves functional capacity without inducing systemic inflammation in claudicants. European Journal of Vascular Surgery 27:201–209

Breit R, van der Wall H 2004 Transcutaneous electrical nerve stimulation for postoperative pain relief after total knee arthroplasty. Journal of Arthroplasty 19:45–48

Brosseau L, Yonge K, Marchand S et al 2002 Efficacy of transcutaneous electrical nerve stimulation (TENS) for rheumatoid arthritis: a systematic review. Physical Therapy Review 7:199–208

Brosseau L, Yonge K, Marchand S et al 2004 Efficacy of transcutaneous electrical nerve stimulation for osteoarthritis of the lower extremities: a meta-analysis. Physical Therapy Review 9:213–233

Carroll D, Tramer M, McQuay H et al 1997 Transcutaneous electrical nerve stimulation in labour pain: a systemic review. British Journal of Obstetrics and Gynaecology 104:169–175

Cheing G, Hui-Chan C, Chan K M 2002 Does four weeks of TENS and/or isometric exercise produce cumulative reduction of osteoarthritic knee pain? Pain Reviews 9:141–151

Chesterton L S, Foster N E, Wright C C et al 2003 Effects of TENS frequency, intensity and stimulation site parameter manipulation on pressure pain thresholds in healthy subjects. Pain 106:73–80

Chiu T, Hui-Chan C, Cheing G 2005 A randomized clinical trial of TENS and exercise for patients with chronic neck pain. Clinical Rehabilitation 19:850–860

Johnson M 2002 Transcutaneous electrical nerve stimulation (TENS). In: Kitchen S (ed) Electrotherapy: evidence-based practice, 11th edn. Churchill Livingstone, Edinburgh, p 259–286

Johnson M I 1998 Acupuncture-like transcutaneous electrical nerve stimulation (AL-TENS) in the management of pain. Physical Therapy Review 3:73–93

Kaplan B, Rabinerson D, Lurie S et al 1998 Transcutaneous electrical nerve stimulation (TENS) for adjuvant pain-relief during labour and delivery. International Journal of Gynecology and Obstetrics 60:251–255

Kaye V, Brandstater M E 2005 Transcutaneous electrical nerve stimulation. Online. Available: http://www.emedicine.com/pmr/topic206.htm

Khadilkar A, Milne S, Brosseau L et al 2005 Transcutaneous electrical nerve stimulation for the treatment of chronic low back pain: A systematic review. Spine 30:2657–2666

Köke A J A, Schouten J S A G, Lamerichs-Geelen M J H et al 2004 Pain reducing effect of three types of transcutaneous electrical nerve stimulation in patients with chronic pain: a randomized crossover trial. Pain 108:36–42

Miller L, Mattison P, Paul L, Wood L 2005 The effects of transcutaneous electrical nerve stimulation on spasticity. Physical Therapy Review 10:201–208

Moore S R, Shurman J 1997 Combined neuromuscular electrical stimulation and transcutaneous electrical nerve stimulation for treatment of chronic back pain: a double-blind, repeated measures comparison. Archives of Physical Medical Rehabilitation 78:55–60

Ng M M L, Leung M C P, Poon D M Y 2003 The effects of electro-acupuncture and transcutaneous electrical nerve stimulation on patients with painful osteoarthritic knees: A randomized controlled trial with follow-up evaluation. Journal of Alternative and Complementary Medicine 9:641–648

Robertson V, Ward A, Low J et al 2006 Electrotherapy explained: principles and practice, 4th edn. Elsevier Science, Oxford

Sluka K A, Walsh D 2003 Transcutaneous electrical nerve stimulation: basic science mechanisms and clinical effectiveness. Journal of Pain 4:109–121

Walsh D M 1996 Transcutaneous electrical nerve stimulation and acupuncture points. Complementary Therapies in Medicine 4:133–137

Wilson I, Lowe-Strong A S, Walsh D M 2002 Evidence for transcutaneous electrical nerve stimulation in the management of low back pain? Physical Therapy Review 7:259–265

Yozbatiran N, Donmez N, Bozan O 2006 Electrical stimulation of the wrist and fingers for sensory and functional recovery in acute hemiplegia. Clinical Rehabilitation 20:4–11

CHAPTER 6

Neuromuscular electrical stimulation

PRODUCTION

Neuromuscular electrical stimulation (NMES) is a battery operated pulse generator that sends electrical impulses via the electrodes through the skin to the motor point or muscle belly. The wave form is a biphasic, asymmetrical square wave (Robertson et al 2006, Howe & Trevor 2002).

EQUIPMENT

NMES machine
Battery
Self adhesive electrodes (2 or 4)
Leads
Neurotips for pin-prick (sharp/blunt) testing.

APPLICATION

1. Identify the area of application and ensure that it is clean.
2. Check for any contraindications.
3. Perform a pin-prick (sharp/blunt) test.
4. Place the electrodes either over the motor point of the muscle or either end of the muscle belly.
5. Attach the leads to the machine.
6. Set the desired frequency, pulse duration and on/off time.
7. Turn up the intensity until a suitable muscle contraction occurs.
8. Start the timer; usual treatment time is 15 min.
9. At the end of the treatment, turn the machine off and remove the electrodes, checking the skin for any signs of adverse reactions.
10. The patient may have to be taught how to do this as NMES treatment is optimal several times a day, depending on the condition.

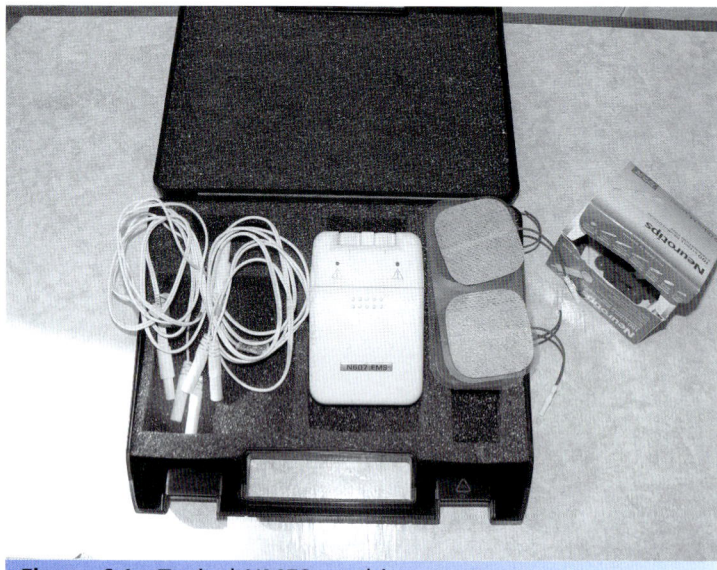

Figure 6.1 Typical NMES machine.

ADAPTATIONS

There are machines available with pre-set programme chips, which will automatically set the parameters of the treatment according to the diagnosis.

Other machines available are functional electrical stimulators (FES), which are used in conjunction with normal functional activities (Fig. 6.4).

APPLICATIONS OF NMES

To increase muscle strength
To promote continence
To maintain or improve range of movement (ROM)
To increase and improve the blood supply to the muscle in cases of intermittent claudication
To help alleviate the changes of muscle tone as appropriate in muscle spasm and spasticity
To prevent disuse atrophy, e.g. rheumatoid arthritis.

CONDITIONS KNOWN TO RESPOND TO NMES

1. Urinary and rectal incontinence
2. Chronic neurological conditions to decrease spasticity, to strengthen muscle and promote higher levels of activity

Neuromuscular electrical stimulation 105

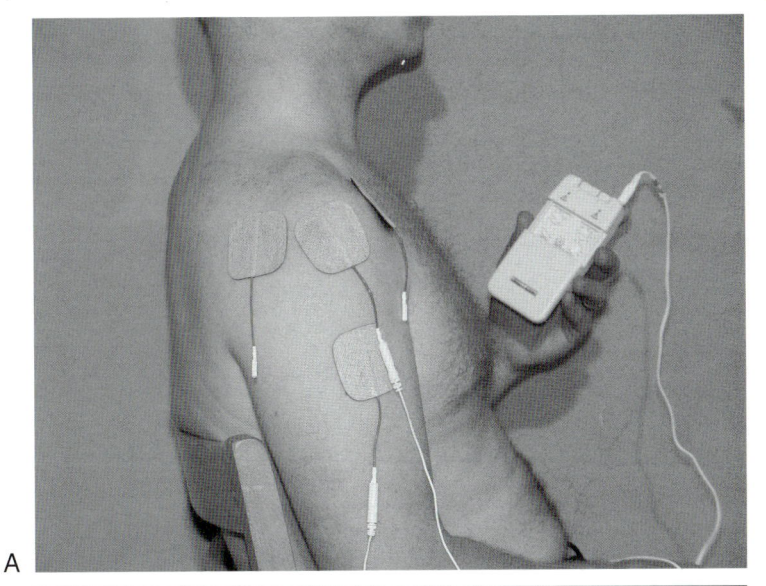

Figure 6.2 (A,B) NMES applied to the deltoid muscle. Two electrodes are placed on either end of the muscle belly of the middle fibres of deltoid. The other two electrodes are placed on the upper attachments of the anterior and posterior fibres of deltoid.

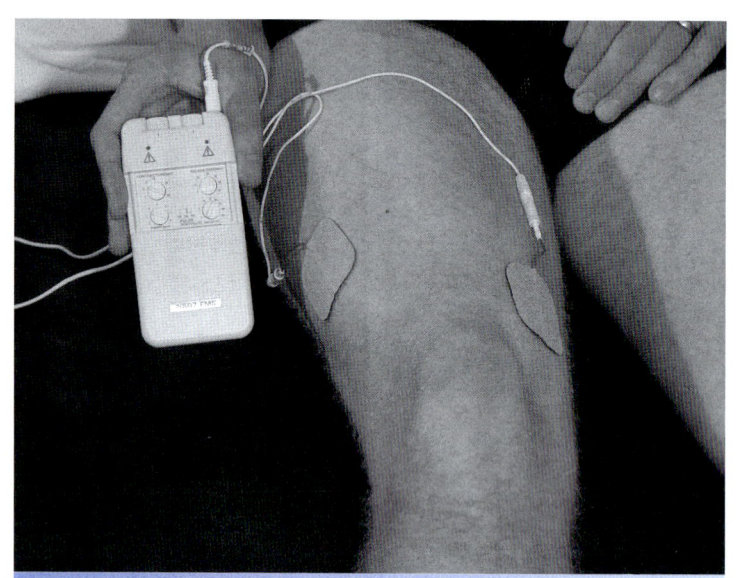

Figure 6.3 NMES applied to the quadriceps muscle. One electrode is on the motor point of vastus medialis and the other electrode is on the motor point of vastus lateralis.

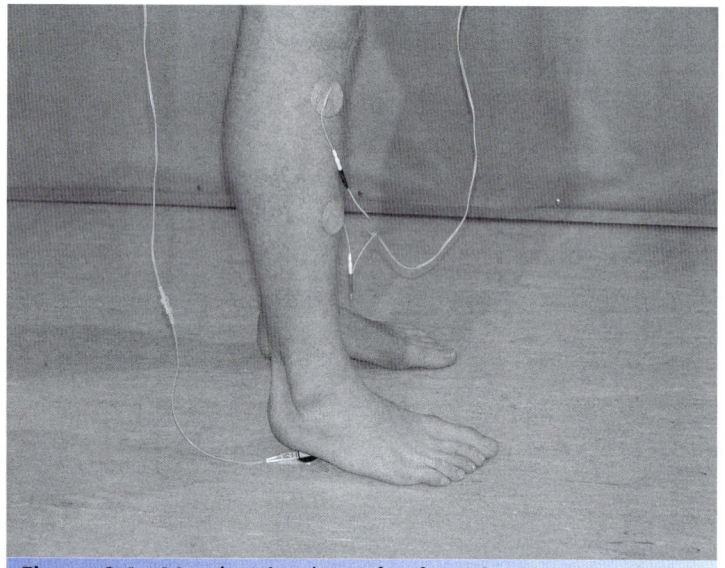

Figure 6.4 Muscle stimulator for foot drop. One electrode can be placed over the common peroneal nerve (head of fibula) and the other on the motor point of tibialis anterior. Raising the heel off the switch (under the heel) activates the stimulation of tibialis anterior and the foot is then able to clear the floor when taking a step.

3. Peripheral nerve lesions, including brachial plexus and Bell's palsy
4. Arthritis for muscle atrophy and pain relief.

Contraindications
Patients fitted with a demand style pacemaker
Over or near the uterus during pregnancy
During pregnancy
Undiagnosed pain
Peripheral vascular disease
Neoplastic tissue
After deep X-ray therapy; devitalised skin
Patients who cannot understand instructions.

Do not apply the electrodes to the following areas:
Mouth
Carotid sinus
Broken skin
Anaesthetised skin
The abdomen during pregnancy
Near the eyes
Over the trachea or larynx.

(See Robertson et al 2006, Howe & Trevor 2002.)

MOTOR POINTS

The motor point is the point where the motor nerve enters the muscle. This is usually found at the junction of the proximal third with the distal two-thirds of the muscle belly.

108 PRACTICAL ELECTROTHERAPY

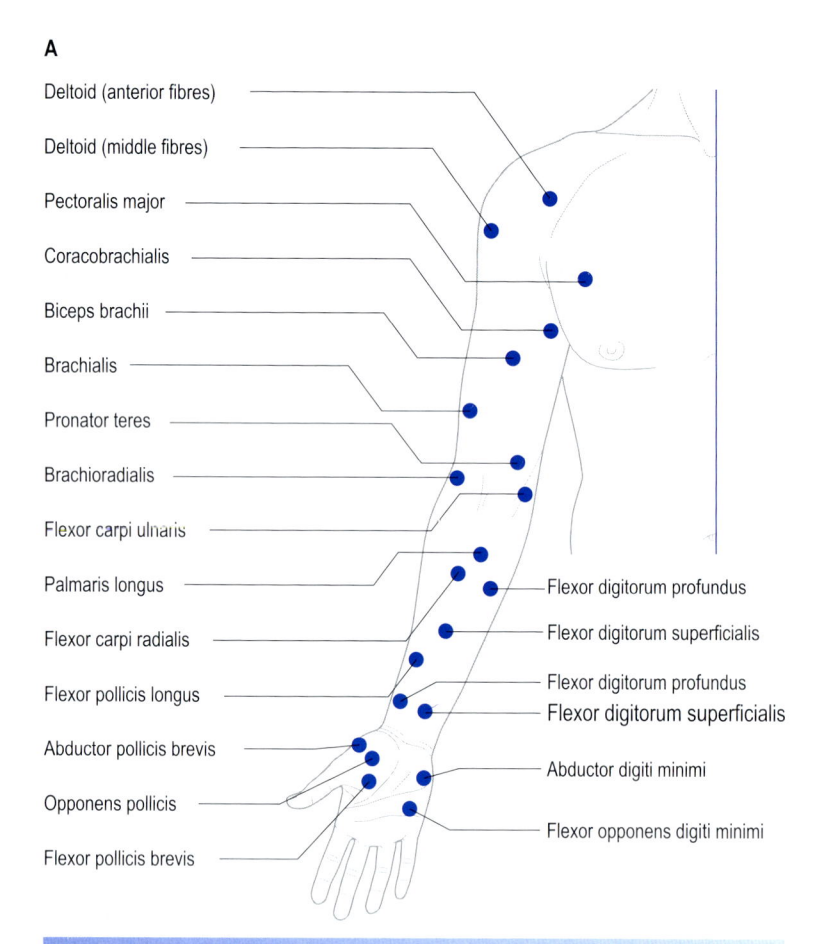

A

- Deltoid (anterior fibres)
- Deltoid (middle fibres)
- Pectoralis major
- Coracobrachialis
- Biceps brachii
- Brachialis
- Pronator teres
- Brachioradialis
- Flexor carpi ulnaris
- Palmaris longus
- Flexor carpi radialis
- Flexor pollicis longus
- Abductor pollicis brevis
- Opponens pollicis
- Flexor pollicis brevis

- Flexor digitorum profundus
- Flexor digitorum superficialis
- Flexor digitorum profundus
- Flexor digitorum superficialis
- Abductor digiti minimi
- Flexor opponens digiti minimi

Figure 6.5 Body chart of motor points.

Neuromuscular electrical stimulation 109

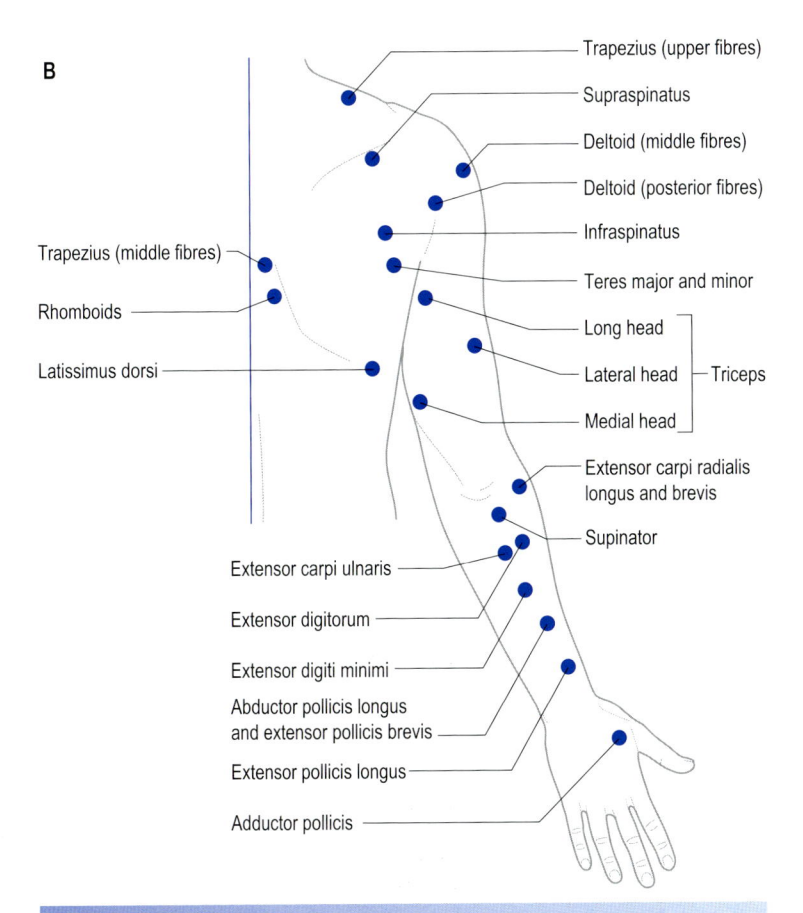

B

- Trapezius (upper fibres)
- Supraspinatus
- Deltoid (middle fibres)
- Deltoid (posterior fibres)
- Infraspinatus
- Trapezius (middle fibres)
- Teres major and minor
- Rhomboids
- Long head
- Latissimus dorsi
- Lateral head ⎤
- Medial head ⎦ Triceps
- Extensor carpi radialis longus and brevis
- Supinator
- Extensor carpi ulnaris
- Extensor digitorum
- Extensor digiti minimi
- Abductor pollicis longus and extensor pollicis brevis
- Extensor pollicis longus
- Adductor pollicis

Figure 6.5, cont'd

C

- Sartorius
- Tensor fasciae latae
- Rectus femoris
- Vastus lateralis
- Vastus medialis
- Peroneus longus
- Tibialis anterior
- Extensor digitorum longus
- Peroneus brevis
- Extensor hallucis longus
- Extensor digitorum brevis

D

- Gluteus medius and minimus
- Gluteus maximus
- Biceps femoris
- Semimembranosus and semitendinosus
- Medial head ⎤
- Lateral head ⎦ Gastrocnemius
- Soleus
- Flexor digitorum longus
- Flexor hallucis longus
- Tibialis posterior

Figure 6.5, cont'd

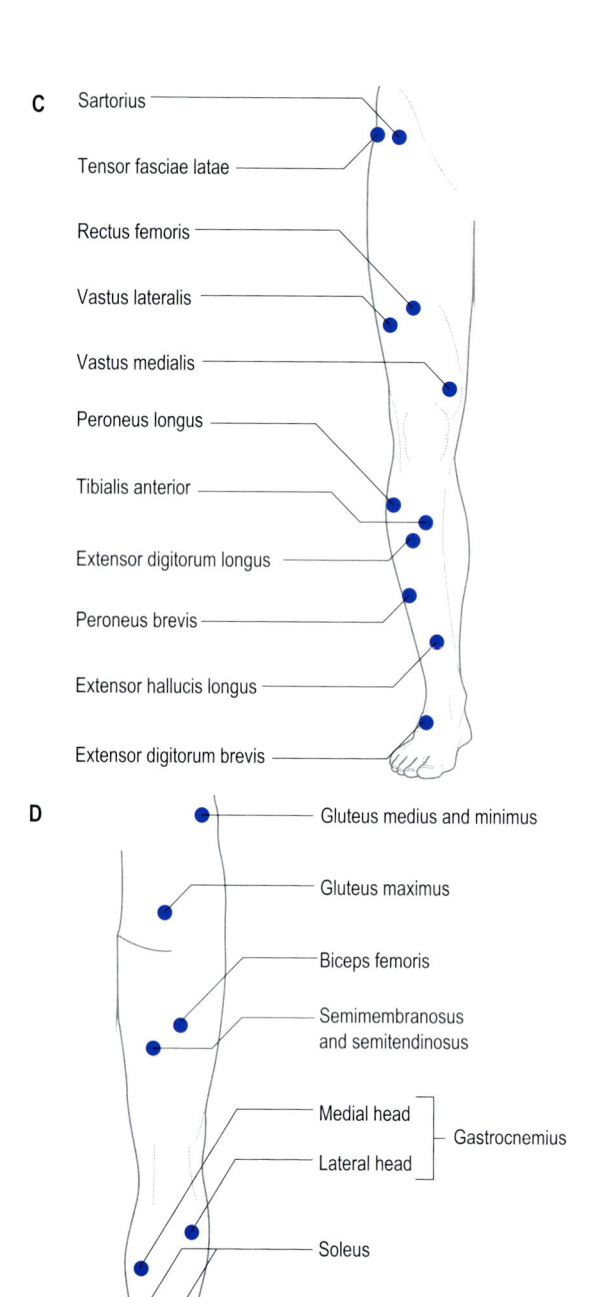

Notes

112 PRACTICAL ELECTROTHERAPY

Treatment record

Table 6.1 *OBSERVATIONAL/REFLECTIVE CHECKLIST*

	Observation	Y/N	Comments
Introduction	Did the therapist introduce him/herself?	☐	☐
	Was an explanation of the procedure given?	☐	☐
	Was the explanation clear and succinct?	☐	☐
	Were the possible dangers highlighted?	☐	☐
	Was consent obtained?	☐	☐
Comfort and safety	Was the patient comfortable?	☐	☐
	Was the therapist's posture compromised?	☐	☐
	Was the position safe for both parties?	☐	☐
	Was the modality applied with due care and attention?	☐	☐
Technique	Were the contraindications checked?	☐	☐
	Were the appropriate tests performed prior to treatment?	☐	☐
	Was an explanation of the physiological effects of the technique offered to the patient?	☐	☐
	Was this explanation accurate?	☐	☐
	Was the technique/modality applied correctly?	☐	☐
	Were the correct times and settings used?	☐	☐
	Was the skin checked after the treatment for adverse effects?	☐	☐

Table 6.2 SUMMARY OF STUDIES INVESTIGATING THE EFFECTIVENESS OF NEUROMUSCULAR ELECTRICAL STIMULATION (NMES)

Authors	Aim of study	Numbers	Methods	Assessment	Results
Ada & Foongchomcheay (2002)	To examine the efficacy of surface electrical stimulation for the prevention or reduction of shoulder subluxation after stroke.	Seven studies were reviewed by the authors.	The authors undertook a systematic search of the literature. Seven studies, randomised controlled trials (RCTs), were reviewed by the authors.		The authors conclude that early application of electrical stimulation applied in a way that produces a motor response in deltoid and supraspinatus muscles is effective in preventing shoulder subluxation.
Avramidis et al (2003)	To investigate the possible effect of electrical muscle stimulation (EMS) of the vastus medialis on the walking speed, Hospital for Special Surgery (HSS) knee score and Physiological Cost Index (PCI) of patients after total knee arthroplasty (TKA).	30 patients, undergoing TKA, were assigned to two groups.	The Treatment Group: (15 subjects) received conventional treatment and EMS to vastus medialis (frequency of 40 Hz, pulse width of 300 µs, 8 s on/off, maximum tolerable intensity for 2 h) twice daily, for 6 weeks postoperatively. The Control Group: (15 subjects) received conventional treatment.	All participants were assessed preoperatively, at 6 weeks and 12 weeks for walking speed, PCI and HSS knee score.	There was a significant increase in walking speed in the treatment group compared with the control group at both 6 weeks ($p = 0.0002$) and 12 weeks ($p = 0.0001$). There was no significant difference between treatment and control groups for PCI or HSS knee score.

Authors	Aim of study	Numbers	Methods	Assessment	Results
Banerjee et al (2005)	To investigate the effects of prolonged use of electrical muscle stimulation (EMS) on physical fitness and body weight in healthy sedentary adults.	15 healthy sedentary adults participated in a crossover study and were randomly assigned to two groups.	*Group A*: received a 6-week training programme of EMS to the quadriceps, hamstrings, gluteal and calf muscles (frequency of 10 Hz, maximum output 300 mA) for 1 h/day, 5 days/week. They then had a 2-week washout period followed by a 6-week period where they maintained their habitual activity level. *Group B*: maintained their habitual activity level for 6 weeks, followed by a 2-week washout period and then a 6-week EMS programme.	Exercise capacity (peak oxygen consumption, VO_2) was evaluated using a modified Bruce treadmill exercise test and a 6 min walk distance test. Isometric quadriceps muscle strength was assessed using a dynamometer. The body mass index (BMI) was calculated.	Following 6 weeks of EMS, there was a significant increase in peak oxygen consumption (VO_2) ($p < 0.05$), walking distance ($p < 0.005$) and quadriceps strength ($p < 0.005$).

PRACTICAL ELECTROTHERAPY

Authors	Aim of study	Numbers	Methods	Assessment	Results
Blowman et al (1991)	To assess the efficacy of neuromuscular stimulation (NMS) and pelvic floor exercises, compared with pelvic floor exercises alone, in the treatment of genuine stress incontinence (GSI).	14 patients with GSI were randomly assigned to two groups.	*Group 1:* (7 subjects) received pelvic floor exercises and neutrophic stimulation (NTS) (frequency of 10 Hz, pulse width 80 µs, 4 s on/off for 60 min) applied daily for 4 weeks. They also received NTS treatment for a further 2 weeks, with a frequency of 35 Hz for 15 min daily. *Group 2:* (7 subjects) received pelvic floor exercise and placebo stimulation.	Patients were assessed by perineometer readings and reduced episodes of incontinence.	The study demonstrated the combined effectiveness of NTS and pelvic floor exercises.
Bo et al (1999)	To compare the effect of pelvic floor exercises, electrical stimulation, vaginal cones and no treatment for genuine stress incontinence (GSI).	107 patients with GSI were randomly assigned to four groups.	*Group 1:* (25 subjects) received pelvic floor muscle training. *Group 2:* (25 subjects) received vaginal electrical stimulation (frequency 50 Hz, pulse width 200 µs, on: 0.5–10 s, off: 0–30 s, maximum tolerable intensity for 30 min) daily for 6 months.	Patients were assessed using a pad test and the severity of the condition using a 5-point scale.	Pelvic floor exercises were more effective than electrical stimulation, vaginal cones and no treatment, for women with GSI.

Authors	Aim of study	Numbers	Methods	Assessment	Results
			Group 3: (27 subjects) received vaginal cone for 20 min a day. Group 4: (30 subjects) received no treatment.		
Dobšák et al (2006)	To evaluate the effects of low-frequency electrical stimulation (LFES) on muscle strength and blood supply in patients with severe grades of chronic heart failure (CHF).	15 patients with advanced grades of CHF participated in the study.	All participants received low-frequency electrical stimulation (frequency of 10 Hz, pulse width of 200 μs, 20 s on/off, a maximal stimulation amplitude of 60 mA) to the quadriceps and calf muscles for 60 min a day, 7 days/week for 6 weeks.	Maximal quadriceps muscle strength was measured weekly using an isometric dynamometer. Blood flow velocity (BFV) was measured by Doppler assessment at baseline and after 6 weeks of LFES. A modified quality of life (QOL) questionnaire was used.	After 6 weeks of LFES, there was a significant increase in muscle strength ($p < 0.001$) and isokinetic peak torque ($p < 0.01$). BFV also showed a significant increase ($p < 0.05$).
Gaines et al (2004)	To examine the short-and long-term effects of a home-based, 12-week neuromuscular	38 elderly patients with OA of the knee were randomly assigned to a treatment or an education group.	Group 1: (20 subjects) received the Arthritis Self-Help Course plus NMES (frequency 50 Hz, ramp 3 s, 10 s on/50 s off) to vastus medialis	Patients' pain was assessed 15 min before treatment and 15 min after treatment, using the NMES Pain Diary (by numerical pain	There was a significant decline of 22% in pain 15 min after NMES, compared with before NMES ($p < 0.001$), measured by

Authors	Aim of study	Numbers	Methods	Assessment	Results
	electrical stimulation (NMES) of the quadriceps femoris to decrease arthritic knee pain in older adults with osteoarthritis (OA) of the knee.		and vastus lateralis, for 15 min/day, 3 days a week for 12 weeks. The stimulator was set to induce a muscle contraction that was a 10–20% maximum voluntary contraction for 4 weeks, 20–30% over the next 4 weeks and 30–40% over the last 4 weeks. *Group 2:* (18 subjects) received the Arthritis Self-Help Course (a 12-h community-based education course.	scale of 1–10). Knee pain was assessed at weeks 0, 4, 8, 12 and 16 with the McGill Pain Questionnaire and the Arthritis Impact Measurement Scale.	the Pain Diary. Both the NMES and education only group showed a non-significant decline in pain from baseline to post-intervention, measured by the McGill Pain Questionnaire. The Arthritis Impact Measurement Scale showed a non-significant increase (7%) in pain for the NMES group and a significant increase (66%) in pain for the education-only group. The authors conclude that there was an immediate decline in arthritic knee pain when NMES was used only 15 min/day, 3 days a week with parameters set for muscle strengthening.

Authors	Aim of study	Numbers	Methods	Assessment	Results
Knight et al (1998)	To evaluate the effectiveness of clinic and home electrical stimulation, in combination with individually planned pelvic floor exercises (PFE) and biofeedback, in the treatment of genuine stress incontinence (GSI).	70 patients with GSI were randomly assigned to three groups.	*Group 1:* (21 subjects) received PFE and biofeedback for 6 months. *Group 2:* (25 subjects) received PFE and low-intensity neuromuscular stimulation (frequency 10 Hz (occasional 35 Hz burst), pulse width 200 μs, 5 s on/off, low intensity to be used at night) for 6 months at home. *Group 3:* (24 subjects) received PFE and acute maximal vaginal electrical stimulation (frequency 35 Hz, pulse width 250 μs, 5 s on/off, maximal intensity for 30 min) 16 sessions in a clinic.	Patients were assessed using: 1. A 7-day frequency chart. 2. Pad testing. 3. Perineometry. 4. Subjective assessment.	57 women completed the trial, which demonstrated that correctly taught pelvic floor exercises, combined with biofeedback, were an effective treatment of patients with GSI. For patients presenting with very weak pelvic floor muscles, the addition of acute maximal electrical stimulation may provide a better treatment outcome.

Authors	Aim of study	Numbers	Methods	Assessment	Results
Lewek et al (2001)	To evaluate the effectiveness of electrical stimulation to increase quadriceps femoris muscle force in an elderly patient following a total knee arthroplasty (TKA).	A case study on an elderly patient following TKA.	This is a case report describing the use of NMES, in addition to a volitional strength training programme to enhance quadriceps femoris muscle force in an elderly patient following total knee arthroplasty (TKA). The electrical stimulator produced an alternating current, triangular wave at 2500 Hz with frequencies ranging from 40 to 75 bursts (Hz) per second. Time on/off was 10/50 s with a 3 second ramp time. 10 contractions were performed. The patient received 18 treatments. The patient was able to return to independent activities of daily living and recreational activities.		

Authors	Aim of study	Numbers	Methods	Assessment	Results
Livesley (1992)	To investigate the effects of electrical neuromuscular stimulation on functional performance in patients with multiple sclerosis (MS).	39 patients with MS were randomly assigned to two groups.	*Group 1:* (20 subjects) received electrical stimulation to the right and left quadriceps and hamstring muscles, 5 times a week for 6 weeks. The programme consisted of stimulation at 3 Hz for 2 min, 10 Hz for 5 min and 35 Hz for 5 min, pulse width of 200 μs and 4 s on/off. *Group 2:* (19 patients) received sham electrical stimulation.	Patients were assessed for passive range of movement, strength of active movement, functional ability and subjective opinion of their condition, on entry to the trial, weekly for 6 weeks and at 3 months after completion of the trial.	The electrical stimulator made no significant difference in the measured parameters of the treatment group compared with the control group.
Moore & Shurman (1997)	To evaluate the use of neuromuscular electrical nerve stimulation (NMES) and combined NMES and TENS for the management of chronic back pain.	24 patients with chronic back pain each received four different interventions, randomly allocated.	1. TENS (frequency 100 Hz, pulse width 100 μs, amplitude producing a comfortable tingling sensation) to the low back for 5 consecutive hours/day for 2 consecutive days.	Each participant completed the Present Pain Intensity (PPI) portion of the McGill Pain Questionnaire and a visual analogue scale (VAS) before and after each treatment.	Combined treatment, TENS and NMES each produced significant pre-treatment to post-treatment reductions in PPI and VAS scores. Combined treatment was superior to both

Authors	Aim of study	Numbers	Methods	Assessment	Results
			2. NMES (frequency 70 Hz, pulse width 200 μs, on/off – 5/15 s, amplitude producing a strong and perceptible contraction of the muscles) to the back. They received three, 10 min periods of stimulation over a 5-h period, for 2 consecutive days. 3. Combined TENS/NMES (same parameters as above) to the back. They received, alternatively one 10 min and one 20 min period of NMES with three periods of TENS stimulation over a 5-h period, for 2 consecutive days. 4. Placebo TENS for 5-h/day for 2 consecutive days. There was a 2-day hiatus period between each intervention to minimise carry-over effects.		TENS and NMES for pain reduction and pain relief. The authors conclude that a regimen of TENS and NMES may be a valuable adjunct in the management of chronic back pain.

Authors	Aim of study	Numbers	Methods	Assessment	Results
Neder et al (2002)	To evaluate the potential for neuromuscular electrical stimulation (NMES) to improve peripheral muscle function, and to evaluate the impact of any such changes on exercise tolerance and health related quality of life of patients with advanced chronic obstructive pulmonary disease (COPD).	15 patients with COPD participated in a crossover study and were randomly assigned to two groups.	*Group 1:* (9 subjects) received NMES (frequency 50 Hz, pulse width 300–400 μs, on/off: 10–30 s, at the highest tolerable intensity for 30 min) 5 times per week for 6 weeks. *Group 2:* (6 subjects) received 6 weeks NMES after a 6-week control period.	Group 1 subjects were assessed before and after NMES. Group 2 subjects were assessed before and after the 6 weeks control period and after the 6 weeks NMES. Patients were assessed using a Chronic Respiratory Disease Questionnaire (CRDQ) for quality of life, body composition, pulmonary function tests, cardiopulmonary exercise tests and quadriceps strength and endurance.	The NMES training programme was associated with significant improvements in muscle function, maximal and endurance exercise tolerance and the dyspnoea domain of the CRDQ.
Pfeifer et al (1997)	To investigate two methods of strengthening the triceps surae at 60% maximal isometric torque, comparing electrical stimulation and volitional isometric contractions.	18 elderly, healthy subjects were assigned to two groups.	*Group 1:* (10 subjects) received electrical stimulation (carrier frequency of 2500 Hz, frequency 80 Hz, 15 s contraction, 50 s rest and 10 contractions each session), 3 times per week for 6 weeks.	Muscle torque of the triceps surae (calf muscles) was assessed.	Both forms of strengthening programme resulted in a significant increase in isometric torque.

Authors	Aim of study	Numbers	Methods	Assessment	Results
			Group 2: (8 subjects) performed 10 contractions each session (15 s contraction, 50 s rest), 3 times per week for 6 weeks.		
Robertson & Ward (2002)	To examine the effect of electrical stimulation of the vastus medialis muscle on stiffness, pain and function for a patient with delayed functional progress following lateral patellar retinacular release.	A single case study.	The patient received electrical stimulation (frequency of 55 Hz–70 Hz, pulse duration 300 μs, on/off: 6 s/3 s, intensity 45 mA–75 mA) to the vastus medialis, delivering 171–360 contractions/day, 7 days a week for a total of 33 days.	Strength of vastus medialis was tested isometrically. The ability to ascend and descend stairs unaided was measured and the ability to hop on the left leg unassisted was assessed. The patient filled in a daily visual analogue score (VAS) for pain and stiffness.	Stiffness was rapidly reduced and after 8 days, the patient could ascend four stairs unaided. After 23 days, the patient could ascend and descend 22 stairs. After 37 days, the patient could perform five consecutive hops, unsupported.
Sand et al (1995)	To determine the efficacy of transvaginal electrical stimulation in treating genuine stress incontinence (GSI).	52 women with GSI were randomly assigned to an active group or a control (sham) group.	The Active Group: (35 subjects) received transvaginal electrical stimulation. The Control Group: (17 subjects) received 'sham' stimulation.	Measurements assessed were weekly and daily voiding diaries, urodynamic testing (including pad test) and pelvic floor muscle strength (using a perineometer).	The authors concluded that transvaginal pelvic floor electrical stimulation was a safe and effective treatment for GSI.

Authors	Aim of study	Numbers	Methods	Assessment	Results
Snyder-Mackler et al (1994)	To investigate the use of electrical stimulation to enhance the recovery of quadriceps femoris muscle force production on patients following anterior cruciate ligament (ACL) reconstruction.	52 patients, having undergone ACL reconstruction were assigned to two groups.	*Group 1:* (31 subjects) received electrical stimulation (2500 Hz, triangular alternating current at a burst rate of 75 Hz, an intensity (mA) set at the patient's maximally tolerated level for 15 contractions each session), 3 times per week for 4 weeks. *Group 2:* (21 subjects) received electrical stimulation (frequency 55 Hz, pulse width of 300 µs, 15 s on/50 s off, maximal intensity (>50 mA) for 15 min), 4 times/day, 5 days per week for 4 weeks.	The knee extension torque produced from the electrically elicited quadriceps femoris muscle contraction was monitored and this torque was expressed as a percentage of the uninvolved quadriceps femoris muscles' maximal contraction force.	The subjects training with the clinical stimulator trained at higher intensities than those training with the battery-powered stimulator, resulting in a higher quadriceps femoris muscle torque.

Authors	Aim of study	Numbers	Methods	Assessment	Results
Stevens et al (2004)	To assess the effect of high-intensity neuromuscular electrical stimulation (NMES) on quadriceps strength and voluntary activation following total knee arthroplasty (TKA).	Eight patients with primary bilateral total knee replacements were assigned to one of two interventions.	*Group 1:* (5 subjects) participated in a voluntary exercise programme for both knees and NMES (delivering an alternating current of 2500 Hz, modulated at 50 Hz, on/off, 10/80 s at a maximum tolerable intensity) for the weaker knee. *Group 2:* (3 subjects) participated in a voluntary exercise programme for both knees (quadriceps). All the patients attended clinic 3 times a week for 6 weeks (18 treatments).	Each participant had their quadriceps strength and voluntary muscle activation tested using an isokinetic dynamometer. This was repeatedly assessed up to 6 months after surgery.	At 6 months, the weak NMES-treated legs of four out of the five patients had surpassed the strength of the contralateral leg. The authors conclude that the study supports the use of high-intensity NMES to promote quadriceps strength gains following TKA.

Table 6.3 **SUMMARY OF STUDIES INVESTIGATING THE EFFECTIVENESS OF FUNCTIONAL ELECTRICAL STIMULATION (FES)**

Authors	Aim of study	Numbers	Methods	Assessment	Results
Berner et al (2004)	To examine the Handmaster electrical stimulation (ES) treatment as an integral part of the rehabilitation process and to evaluate its effect on the functional rehabilitation of acute cerebrovascular accident (CVA) elderly patients.	22 subjects with CVA participated in the study.	All the patients received daily rehabilitation. In addition, they all received electrical stimulation (frequencies of 18 Hz and 36 Hz, from 10 to 60 min) twice daily for 3 weeks. After a 3-week break from ES, a group of nine subjects received a further 3-week course of ES, the remaining 13 subjects continued only with their rehabilitation programme.	Functional assessment was evaluated before and after intervention. Measurements included: range of movement (ROM) of the upper limb, manual dexterity tests and the functional independence measure (FIM).	All 22 subjects showed a significant improvement in ROM, manual dexterity and FIM after the first 3-week treatment. After the two periods of electrical treatment, the nine subjects showed significant improvement in ROM and manual dexterity. The authors conclude that the Handmaster ES treatment can improve the rehabilitation outcome in elderly patients with sensorimotor deficit caused by CVA.

Authors	Aim of study	Numbers	Methods	Assessment	Results
Chantraine et al (1999)	To determine the influence of functional electrical stimulation (FES) on subluxation and shoulder pain in hemiplegic patients.	120 hemiplegic patients, receiving conventional rehabilitation, were alternately assigned to a control group and a group receiving FES.	*The Treatment Group:* (60 subjects) received FES (pulse width 350 μs, on/off – 1:5, frequency 8 Hz for 90 min, 40 Hz for 30 min and 1 Hz for 10 min) to the shoulder muscles, daily, for 5 weeks. *The Control Group:* (60 subjects) received conventional physiotherapy.	Pain was assessed using the visual analogue scale (VAS). Range of shoulder movement was measured and the level of subluxation (radiologically).	The group receiving FES showed significantly more improvement than the control group in pain relief ($p < 0.01$) and reduction of subluxation ($p < 0.05$). The authors conclude that the FES programme was significantly effective in reducing the severity of subluxation and pain and may possibly have facilitated recovery of the shoulder function in hemiplegic patients.
Glanz et al (1996)	To assess the efficacy of functional electrical stimulation (FES) in the rehabilitation of stroke patients.		The authors undertook a systematic search of the literature. Four studies, RCTs, were reviewed by the authors, who then undertook a meta-analysis.		Pooling from RCTs supports FES as promoting recovery of muscle strength after stroke.

Authors	Aim of study	Numbers	Methods	Assessment	Results
Granat et al (1996)	To assess the orthotic and therapeutic value of the peroneal stimulator (PS) for adult hemiplegic patients.	17 patients with a cerebrovascular accident (CVA) participated in the study.	Each patient received normal physiotherapy treatment for 4 weeks (control period). During the treatment period (4 weeks) they were encouraged to use the PS (frequency 25–50 Hz, pulse width 300 μs and stimulus applied to common peroneal nerve to cause dorsiflexion at the ankle) daily.	Gait was assessed with the patient required to walk over smooth linoleum, carpet and uneven ground. The Barthel Index was applied once during each testing session.	There was a significant orthotic improvement in inversion on all surfaces and for swing symmetry on linoleum. There was a significant improvement in the Barthel Index over the treatment period.
Johnson et al (2004)	To investigate the effect of combined botulinum type A (BTX) and functional electrical stimulation (FES) treatment on spastic drop foot in stroke patients.	18 hemiplegic patients with a spastic drop foot were randomly assigned to two groups.	*The Treatment Group:* (10 subjects) received a normal physiotherapy programme. At the end of a baseline period (4 weeks) they received BTX and began using FES (frequency 40 Hz, pulse width between 30–350 μs, current amplitude up to 100 mA) to stimulate the common peroneal	Walking speed was assessed over a 10 m walkway. The Physical Cost Index (PCI) was also measured along with the walking speed assessment. The Modified Ashworth Scale (MAS) was scored and the Rivermead Motor Assessment (RMA) measured function. The Medical	Walking speed significantly increased for the control group and the treatment group. There was a significant decrease in PCI for the treatment group. There was a significant increase in RMA score in the treatment group. The authors conclude that the study showed

Authors	Aim of study	Numbers	Methods	Assessment	Results
			nerve. This was used for most of the day to aid walking, and continuously for 12 weeks. *The Control Group:* (8 subjects) received a normal physiotherapy programme for the 16-week period.	Outcomes Study 36-Item Short-Form Health survey was also used for assessment.	an improvement in walking speed with patients with a spastic drop foot treated with BTX and FES in combination.
Kim et al (2004)	To compare the effect of functional electrical stimulation (FES) with that of a hinged ankle-foot orthosis (AFO) for assisting foot clearance, gait speed, and endurance and to determine whether there is added benefit in using FES in conjunction with the hinged AFO on patients with incomplete spinal cord injury (SCI).	19 patients with incomplete SCI participated in the study.	Each participant walked along an 8 m walkway under four randomly selected conditions: with an AFO, with FES (electrodes over the common peroneal nerve), with AFO and FES and with no orthosis.	Gait speed, 6-min walking distance, and foot clearance values were compared between conditions.	Gait speed increased with FES and AFO. 6-min walking speed increased with AFO. Foot clearance improved with FES but not with AFO. The authors concluded that the AFO and FES used in combination provided greater benefits in overall gait function than either device alone.

Authors	Aim of study	Numbers	Methods	Assessment	Results
Kottink et al (2004)	This systematic review was carried out to establish the available evidence of the orthotic effect of peroneus nerve stimulation on walking speed.	Eight studies were reviewed by the authors.	The authors undertook a systematic search of the literature. Eight studies fulfilled the selection criteria and were reviewed by the authors.		The authors concluded that FES seems to have a positive orthotic effect on walking speed and the physiological cost index (PCI).
Newsam & Baker (2004)	To compare the maximum voluntary isometric torque (MVIT) and motor unit recruitment of the quadriceps after an electrical stimulation facilitation programme in persons affected by cerebrovascular accident (CVA).	20 patients with a CVA were randomly assigned to a study group and a control group.	*The Study Group:* (10 subjects) received standard physiotherapy and electrical stimulation (frequency 35 Hz, pulse width 220 μs) applied over vastus medialis and vastus lateralis and activated during the stance phase of gait or weight-bearing activities. They received treatment 5 days a week for 3 weeks. *The Control Group:* (10 subjects) received standard physiotherapy 6 days a week for 3 weeks.	Maximum voluntary isometric torque (MVIT) of the hemiparetic knee extensors was measured using an isokinetic dynamometer.	MVIT increased by 77% in patients receiving electrical stimulation, compared with a 31% increase for the control group. The authors concluded that an electrical stimulation programme integrated into weight-bearing activities can significantly increase quadriceps recruitment in persons recovering from a stroke.

Authors	Aim of study	Numbers	Methods	Assessment	Results
Taylor et al (1999)	To assess the clinical effectiveness of the Odstock foot stimulator by analysis of its effect on physiological cost index (PCI) and speed of walking.	151 patients with a dropped foot, due to an upper motor neurone lesion participated in the study.	Each patient received electrical stimulation (frequency 40 Hz, maximum pulse duration of 300 μs, maximum amplitude 80 mA) to the common peroneal nerve and the motor point of the tibialis anterior muscle.	Changes in walking speed and effort of walking, as measured by PCI over a 10-m course was assessed at the initial appointment and 4.5 months later. Walking speed and PCI were measured both with the patient using the stimulator and without the stimulator.	140 patients completed the study. The stroke patients showed a mean increase in walking speed of 27% ($p < 0.01$) and reduction in PCI of 31% ($p < 0.01$) with stimulation and changes of 14% ($p < 0.01$) and 19% ($p < 0.01$), respectively, when not using the stimulator. Multiple sclerosis patients gained similar orthotic benefits. The authors concluded that the use of the stimulator improved walking.

Authors	Aim of study	Numbers	Methods	Assessment	Results
Yan et al (2005)	To investigate whether functional electrical stimulation (FES) combined with a standard rehabilitation (SR) programme was more effective than a SR programme given with placebo stimulation or alone in promoting the recovery of motor function and functional mobility during acute stroke.	41 patients having suffered a stroke participated in the study.	*Group 1*: (13) received standard rehabilitation (SR) and FES (frequency of 30 Hz, pulse width 300 μs, at maximum tolerable intensity for 30 min) applied to the quadriceps, hamstrings, tibialis anterior and medial gastrocnemius. Patients were treated 5 days/week for 3 weeks. *Group 2*: (15) received SR and placebo FES (settings as above but the circuit did not function). Patients were treated for 60 min, 5 days/week for 3 weeks. *Group 3*: (13) received SR only for 60 min, 5 days/week for 3 weeks.	The outcome measurements included the composite spasticity score, maximum voluntary isometric contraction of the ankle dorsiflexors and plantarflexors, and walking ability. Measurements were recorded before treatment, weekly during the 3 weeks of treatment and 8 weeks after the onset of the stroke.	There was a significant reduction in the percentage of composite spasticity score. There was a significant improvement in the ankle dorsiflexion torque. All subjects in the FES group were able to walk after treatment. The authors conclude that 15 sessions of FES, given for 30 min per session plus SR, 5 days/week, improved motor recovery and functional mobility in acute stroke patients.

REFERENCES

Ada L, Foongchomcheay A 2002 Efficacy of electrical stimulation in preventing or reducing subluxation of the shoulder after stroke: a meta-analysis. Australian Journal of Physiotherapy 48:257–267

Avramidis K, Strike P W, Taylor P N et al 2003 Effectiveness of electrical stimulation of the vastus medialis muscle in the rehabilitation of patients after total knee arthroplasty. Archives of Physical Medicine and Rehabilitation 84:1850–1853

Banerjee P, Caulfield B, Crowe L et al 2005 Prolonged electrical muscle stimulation exercise improves strength and aerobic capacity in healthy sedentary adults. Journal of Applied Physiology 99:2307–2311

Berner Y N, Kimchi O L, Spokoiny V et al 2004 The effect of electrical rehabilitation of acute geriatric patients with stroke – a preliminary study. Archives of Gerontology and Geriatrics 39:125–132

Blowman C, Pickles C, Emery S et al 1991 Prospective double blind controlled trial of intensive physiotherapy with and without stimulation of the pelvic floor in the treatment of genuine stress incontinence. Physiotherapy 77:661–664

Bo K, Talseth T, Holme I 1999 Single, blind, randomised controlled trial of pelvic floor exercises, electrical stimulation, vaginal cones, and no treatment in management of genuine stress incontinence in women. British Medical Journal 318:487–493

Chantraine A, Baribeault A, Uebelhart D et al 1999 Shoulder pain and dysfunction in hemiplegia: effects of functional electrical stimulation. Archives of Physical Medicine and Rehabilitation 80:328–331

Dobšák P, Nováková M, Siegelová J et al 2006 Low-frequency electrical stimulation increases muscle strength and improves blood supply in patients with chronic heart failure. Circulation Journal 70:75–82

Gaines J M, Metter E J, Talbot L A 2004 The effect of neuromuscular electrical stimulation on arthritis knee pain in older adults with osteoarthritis of the knee. Applied Nursing Research 17:201–206

Glanz M, Klawansky S, Stason W et al 1996 Functional electrostimulation in post-stroke rehabilitation: a meta-analysis of the randomized controlled trials. Archives of Physical Medicine and Rehabilitation 77:549–553

Granat M H, Maxwell D J, Ferguson A C B et al 1996 Peroneal stimulator: evaluation for the correction of drop foot in hemiplegia. Archives of Physical Medicine and Rehabilitation 77:19–24

Howe T, Trevor M 2002 Low-frequency currents – an introduction. In: Kitchen S (ed) Electrotherapy: evidence-based practice, 11th edn. Churchill Livingstone, Edinburgh, p 233–240

Johnson C A, Burridge J H, Strike P W et al 2004 The effect of combined use of botulinum toxin type A and functional electrical stimulation in the treatment of spastic drop foot after stroke: a preliminary investigation. Archives of Physical Medicine and Rehabilitation 85:902–909

Kim C M, Eng J J, Whittaker M W 2004 Effects of a simple functional electric system and/or a hinged ankle-foot orthosis on walking in persons with incomplete spinal cord injury. Archives of Physical Medicine and Rehabilitation 85:1718–1723

Knight S, Laycock J, Naylor D 1998 Evaluation of neuromuscular electrical stimulation in the treatment of genuine stress incontinence. Physiotherapy 84:61–71

Kottink A I R, Oostendorp L J M, Buurke J H et al 2004 The orthotic effect of functional electrical stimulation on the improvement of walking in stroke patients with a dropped foot: a systematic review. Artificial Organs 28:577–586

Lewek M, Stevens L, Snyder-Mackler L 2001 The use of electrical stimulation to increase quadriceps femoris muscle force in an elderly patient following a total knee arthroplasty. Physical Therapy 81:1565–1571

Livesley E 1992 Effects of electrical neuromuscular stimulation on functional performance in patients with multiple sclerosis. Physiotherapy 78:914–917

Moore S R, Shurman J 1997 Combined neuromuscular electrical stimulation and transcutaneous electrical nerve stimulation for treatment of chronic back pain: a double-blind, repeated measures comparison. Archives of Physical Medicine and Rehabilitation 78:5–60

Neder J A, Sword D, Ward S A et al 2002 Home based neuromuscular electrical stimulation as a new rehabilitative strategy for severely disabled patients with chronic obstructive pulmonary disease (COPD). Thorax 57:333–337

Newsam C J, Baker L L 2004 Effect of an electric stimulation facilitation programme on quadriceps motor unit recruitment after stroke. Archives of Physical Medicine and Rehabilitation 85:2040–2045

Pfeifer A M, Cranfield T, Wagner S et al 1997 Muscle strength: A comparison of electrical stimulation and volitional isometric contractions in adults over 65. Physiotherapy Canada Winter:32–39

Robertson V, Ward A, Low J et al 2006 Electrotherapy explained: principles and practice, 4th edn. Elsevier Science, Oxford

Robertson V J, Ward A R 2002 Vastus medialis electrical stimulation to improve lower extremity function following a lateral patellar retinacular release. Journal of Orthopaedics and Sports Physical Therapy 32:437–443

Sand P K, Richardson D A, Staskin D R et al 1995 Pelvic floor electrical stimulation in the treatment of genuine stress incontinence: A multicenter, placebo-controlled trial. American Journal of Obstetrics and Gynecology 173:72–79

Snyder-Mackler L, Delitto A, Stralka S, Bailey S L 1994 Use of electrical stimulation to enhance recovery of quadriceps femoris muscle force production in patients following anterior cruciate ligament reconstruction. Physical Therapy 74:901–907

Stevens J E, Mizner R L, Snyder-Mackler L 2004 Neuromuscular electrical stimulation for quadriceps muscle strengthening after bilateral total knee arthroplasty: a case series. Journal of Orthopaedic and Sports Physical Therapy 34:21–29

Taylor P N, Burridge J H, Dunkerley A L et al 1999 Clinical use of the Odstock dropped foot stimulator: its effect on the speed and effort of walking. Archives of Physical Medicine and Rehabilitation 80:1577–1583

Yan T, Hui-Chan C W Y, Li L S W 2005 Functional electrical stimulation improves motor recovery of the lower extremity and walking ability of subjects with first acute stroke. Stroke 36:80–85

CHAPTER 7

Interferential therapy

PRODUCTION

Interferential therapy (IFT) is seen as a form of transcutaneous electrical nerve stimulation (TENS). The basic principle of interferential therapy is to pass two medium frequency alternating currents, which are slightly out of phase, through the tissues. Where these currents intersect, a new current is set up, which produces a low-frequency effect, known as the beat frequency. The medium frequency current will pass through the skin more easily, require less electrical energy input to reach the deeper tissues and be much more comfortable than a typical low frequency current. This is due to the resistance (impedance) of the skin being inversely proportional to the frequency of the stimulation (Robertson et al 2006, Palmer & Martin 2002).

EQUIPMENT
IFT machine
Cables
Electrodes
Sponges
Bowl of water
Neurotips to test skin sensation
Velcro straps (to hold the electrodes in position).

APPLICATION TO THE LOW BACK USING SUCTION ELECTRODES
1. Position the patient comfortably in a prone lying position.
2. Re-check for contraindications for treatment.
3. Expose the area required and perform a pin-prick test to the entire area.
4. Turn on the suction machine and insert the damp sponges.

PRACTICAL ELECTROTHERAPY

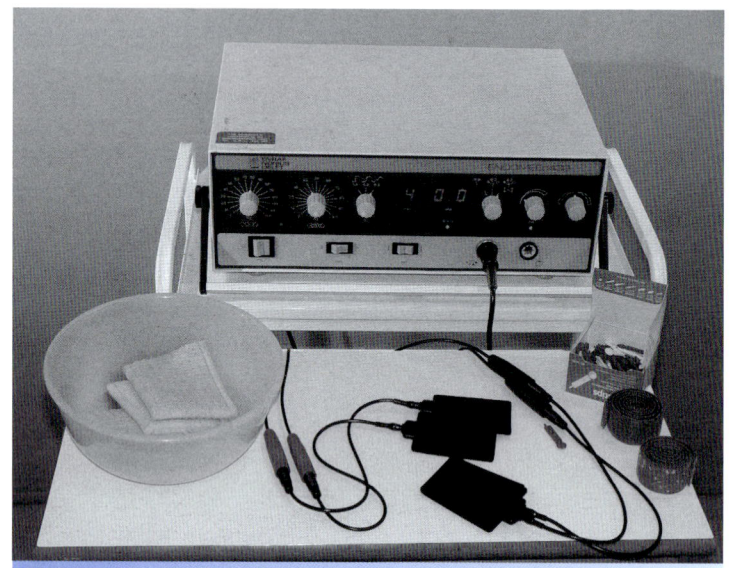

Figure 7.1 An interferential therapy (IFT) machine with malleable electrodes, sponges in warm water, neurotips and Velcro straps.

5. Apply to the area and allow suction to take hold.
6. Ensure the colour of the cables are on opposite corners of the square, i.e. blue to blue on one diagonal and white to white on the opposite diagonal (Fig. 7.2).
7. The electrodes should be placed so that the area to be treated is in the centre. Figure 7.2 shows the area to be treated, where the 'blue' current and the 'white' currents cross.
8. Set the time for treatment: 15–20 min.
9. Set the frequency/frequencies required for treatment and the sweep.
10. Some machines have a rotating vector system allowing for an even distribution of current throughout the tissues.
11. Start the treatment and increase the intensity to a comfortable level for the patient.
12. You may have to increase the intensity after several minutes as the patient will accommodate to the intensity.
13. Once the treatment is over check the area for any adverse effects to treatment.

ADAPTATIONS

Malleable electrodes and suction cups are shown in Figures 7.1 and 7.2, respectively.

Interferential therapy   139

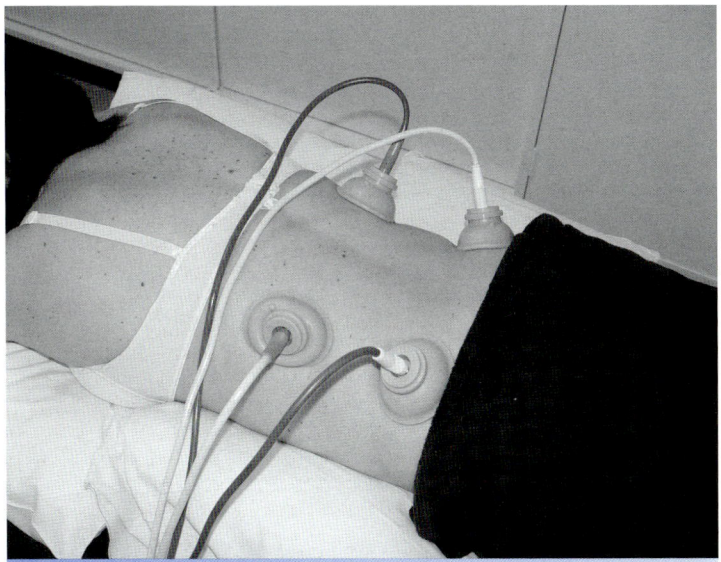

Figure 7.2 IFT to the low back using suction electrodes.

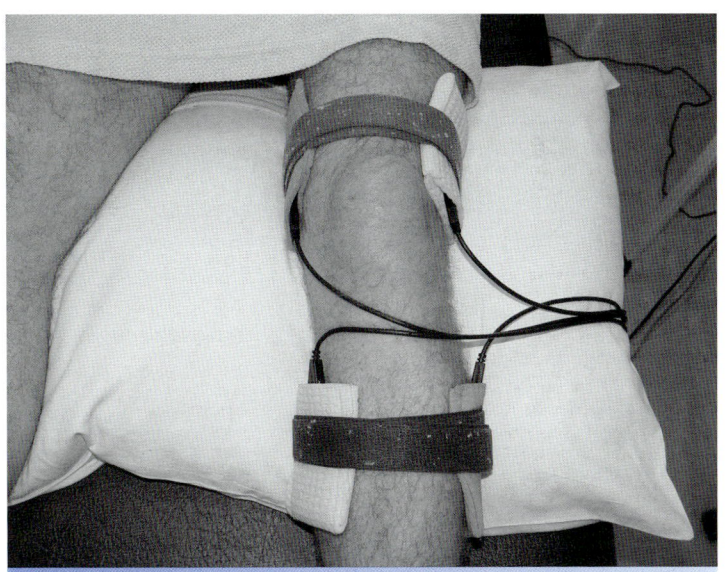

Figure 7.3 IFT to the knee. For illustration purposes, each pair of electrodes have been given a different colour. This shows how the two currents will cross deep in the knee joint.

Physiological effects

The beat frequency produced by the intersecting medium frequency currents will stimulate different tissues according to its frequency.

A broad sweep of frequencies will cover a whole gamut of nerves and thus encompass an array of physiological effects. Table 7.1 is a list of treatment frequencies, the tissues stimulated and the resultant physiological effect.

Contraindications

Very acute inflammation
Any person wearing a cardiac pacemaker
Fever
Thrombosis
Tumours
Over a pregnant uterus.

Table 7.1 TREATMENT FREQUENCIES, TISSUES STIMULATED AND RESULTANT PHYSIOLOGICAL EFFECT

Physiological effect	Frequency	Tissue stimulated
Pain relief	80–120 Hz	Aβ nerve fibres (pain gate)
Pain relief	15 Hz	C-nerve fibres (descending pain suppression)
	10–25 Hz	Aδ and C fibres – PAG → opiate release
Tissue fluid exchange; Muscle contraction	10–150 Hz	Parasympathetic nerves Skeletal muscle
Increased blood supply	0–10 Hz	Sympathetic nerves
Muscle contraction	10–80 Hz 0–10 Hz	Skeletal muscle Smooth muscle
Pelvic floor muscle contraction	1 Hz, 10–40 Hz, 40 Hz	Pelvic floor muscles
Placebo effect	Any frequency	

Interferential therapy

Notes

142 PRACTICAL ELECTROTHERAPY

Treatment record

Table 7.2 *OBSERVATIONAL/REFLECTIVE CHECKLIST*

	Observation	Y/N	Comments
Introduction	Did the therapist introduce him/herself?	☐	☐
	Was an explanation of the procedure given?	☐	☐
	Was the explanation clear and succinct?	☐	☐
	Were the possible dangers highlighted?	☐	☐
	Was consent obtained?	☐	☐
Comfort and safety	Was the patient comfortable?	☐	☐
	Was the therapist's posture compromised?	☐	☐
	Was the position safe for both parties?	☐	☐
	Was the modality applied with due care and attention?	☐	☐
Technique	Were the contraindications checked?	☐	☐
	Were the appropriate tests performed prior to treatment?	☐	☐
	Was an explanation of the physiological effects of the technique offered to the patient?	☐	☐
	Was this explanation accurate?	☐	☐
	Was the technique/modality applied correctly?	☐	☐
	Were the correct times and settings used?	☐	☐
	Was the skin checked after the treatment for adverse effects?	☐	☐

PRACTICAL ELECTROTHERAPY

Table 7.3 SUMMARY OF STUDIES INVESTIGATING THE EFFECTIVENESS OF INTERFERENTIAL THERAPY (IFT)

Authors	Aim of study	Numbers	Methods	Assessment	Results
Adedoyin et al (2002)	To examine the effectiveness of interferential current stimulation (IFT) in modulating osteoarthritis (OA) knee pain.	30 patients with OA of the knee participated in the study and were assigned to two groups.	Group 1: (15 subjects) received IFT (4-pole, frequency 100 Hz for 15 min and 80 Hz for 5 min, at an intensity producing an appreciable sensation) and a mobilising exercise regime, twice weekly for 4 weeks. Group 2: (15 subjects) had the same IFT set-up but the intensity was not turned up and they also received a mobilising exercise regime, twice weekly for 4 weeks.	The patients' pain was assessed using the visual analogue scale (VAS), at initial assessment and after treatment.	There was a significant difference between initial and final pain rating in both groups and a significant difference was found between the two groups.
Christie & Willoughby (1990)	To assess the efficacy of interferential therapy on swelling following open reduction and internal fixation of ankle fractures.	24 patients with ankle fractures were randomly assigned to one of two groups.	Group 1: (12 subjects) received a standard regimen of management and interferential therapy (4 pole, frequency 0–100 Hz, intensity 20 mA, daily for 20 min) for 2–4 days, applied to the ankle. Group 2: (12 subjects) received the standard regimen and sham interferential treatment.	Ankle swelling was measured pre-treatment and post-treatment by performing volumetric measurements.	There was no significant reduction in swelling between the treatment and control groups ($p > 0.05$).

Fourie & Bowerbank (1997)	To establish whether the use of interferential currents (IFCs) reduced the time taken for fractures of the tibia to heal and whether it could lower the incidence of non-union.	208 patients with 227 fractured tibiae, were randomly assigned to two groups.	*Group 1:* (41 subjects) received IFCs via suction electrodes (frequency 10–25 Hz, swing mode 6/6 and an intensity of 25 mA for 30 min) applied daily for 10 treatments. *Group 2:* (35 subjects) suction electrode applied, producing a rhythmical massage effect. Another group (151 subjects) received no treatment.	The outcome measurements used were clinical and radiological union, especially the 'average time until union in weeks'.	The results failed to show any statistically significant effect of treatment on bone healing.
Hurley et al (2001)	To investigate the efficacy of commonly used interferential therapy (IFT) electrode placement techniques for the management of subjects with low back pain: 'painful area' and 'spinal nerve root' in combination with an evidence-based patient education book, *The Back Book*, compared with a control treatment, *The Back Book* alone.	60 subjects with low back pain were randomly assigned to three treatment groups.	*Group 1:* (18 subjects) received IFT (carrier frequency 3.85 kHz, frequency of 140 Hz, pulse duration 130 μs applied at a 'strong but comfortable sensation' for 30 min) to the 'painful area' and *The Back Book*. *Group 2:* (22 subjects) received IFT (treatment parameters identical to the above) to the 'spinal nerve root' and *The Back Book*. *Group 3:* (20 subjects) received *The Back Book* alone.	Each subject was assessed using the McGill Pain Questionnaire (MPQ), the Roland-Morris Disability Questionnaire (RMDQ) and the EurolQol (EQ-5D), pre-treatment, at discharge and at 3 months follow-up.	The results showed that all groups had significant improvements in all outcomes at follow-up. Subjects receiving IFT to the 'spinal nerve' and *The Back Book* displayed both statistically significant ($p = 0.30$) and clinically meaningful reduction in functional disability (RMDQ), compared with the other two groups.

Authors	Aim of study	Numbers	Methods	Assessment	Results
Johnson (1999)	This paper questions some of the beliefs and practices about the clinical use of interferential currents (IFCs).		The author attempts to answer four beliefs about interferential therapy, prevalent in the literature: • Interferential therapy is clinically effective for the management of a variety of ailments. • The physiological and clinical effects of IFCs are mediated by the amplitude modulated wave. • Different frequencies of this amplitude modulated wave will produce different physiological effects. • It is possible to prescribe electrical characteristics of IFC for different medical conditions.		The author says there is little consistent information about the different effects of varying dosages. In fact, there is scanty proof that it works at all.
Johnson & Wilson (1997)	To examine the analgesic effects of 6∧6 and 1/1 swing patterns of interferential currents (IFC) on cold-induced pain in healthy subjects.	15 healthy subjects were randomly allocated to three groups.	Group 1: received active IFC with swing pattern 6∧6 (4 pole, frequency 90–130 Hz, at an intensity which was 'strong but comfortable' for 60 min), applied to the forearm. Group 2: received active IFC with swing pattern 1/1 (same parameters as above). Group 3: received sham IFC treatment (no current).	Measurement of pain threshold and pain intensity rating were taken during six identical 10-min experimental cycles of the cold-induced pain test. The duration of each experiment was 60 min and treatment (either 6∧6, 1/1, or sham) took place during the two 'during treatment' cycles	The authors conclude that the findings of this study suggest that different patterns of IFC may have different analgesic effects.

Authors	Aim of study	Numbers	Methods	Assessment	Results
Lamb & Mani (1994)	To examine methods of assessing arterial and microvascular responses to interferential therapy in healthy subjects.	31 healthy volunteers each undertook three interventions.	Each patient received interferential therapy (4 pole, frequency of 0–30 Hz, 45–90 Hz, and 100–150 Hz on separate occasions, and a current intensity of 35–45 mA for 15 min) applied to the upper calf muscle.		The results suggest that interferential therapy currents can be used to increase arterial and microcirculatory blood flow; and that the response is dose-related.
Laycock & Jerwood (1993) First study	To evaluate, using objective and subjective measures, the effect of transcutaneous, pre-modulated interferential therapy (IFT) on the symptoms of female genuine stress incontinence (GSI).	40 women with GSI were randomly assigned to two groups.	Group 1: (23 subjects) received a course of IFT (bi-polar technique, frequency of 1 Hz, 10–40 Hz, and 40 Hz at maximum current intensity, each for 10 min), completing, on average, 10 treatments. Group 2: (17 subjects) received a course of pelvic floor exercises (PFE) and cones, completing, on average, six sessions.	Pre- and post-treatment evaluation of urine loss was assessed using a standard pad test. Pelvic floor strength was also measured before and after treatment. Frequency/volume charts were completed for 1 week before the first appointment and for 1 week after the final treatment. Patients were assessed subjectively using a 4-point scale.	Subjective assessment showed that 60.9% of the IFT group and 41.2% of the PFE group considered themselves improved or cured. This compares with 43.5% of the IFT group and 58.8% of the PFE group objectively judged to be improved or cured.

Authors	Aim of study	Numbers	Methods	Assessment	Results
Laycock & Jerwood (1993) Second study	To evaluate, using objective and subjective measures, the effect of transcutaneous, pre-modulated interferential therapy (IFT) on the symptoms of female genuine stress incontinence (GSI).	26 women with GSI were randomly assigned to one of two groups.	*Group 1:* (15 subjects) received a course of IFT (bi-polar technique, frequency of 1 Hz, 10–40 Hz, and 40 Hz at a current intensity to produce a 'pins and needles' sensation, each for 10 min), completing on average 10 treatments. *Group 2:* (11 subjects) received placebo IFT (same parameters above but no current).	Pre- and post-treatment evaluation of urine loss was assessed using a standard pad test. Pelvic floor strength was also measured before and after treatment, using a perineometer. Frequency/volume charts were completed for 1 week before the first appointment and for 1 week after the final treatment. Patients were assessed subjectively for frequency using a 6-point scale and for severity using a 5-point scale.	The IFT treatment group demonstrated a significantly greater reduction in pad test weight than the placebo group ($p = 0.0085$). Pelvic floor strength increased significantly for the treatment group ($p = 0.0166$). Subjectively, 33.3% of the IFT group considered themselves improved or cured and 27.3% receiving placebo IFT considered themselves improved or cured.

Authors	Aim of study	Numbers	Methods	Assessment	Results
Noble et al (2000a)	To investigate the effect of various interferential current frequencies upon cutaneous blood flow in humans using laser Doppler flowmetry with concomitant measurement of skin temperature.	50 healthy volunteers were randomly allocated into five groups.	*Group 1:* (10 subjects) control received no suction nor IFT. *Group 2:* (10 subjects) placebo IFT had same set-up as active group but no current delivered. *Group 3:* (10 subjects) received IFT (suction, 4 pole, carrier frequency 4 kHz, pulse duration 125 μs, treatment frequency 10–100 Hz, sweep 6/6, vector, at an intensity producing a 'strong but comfortable' sensation for 15 min) to the right quadriceps femoris muscle. *Group 4:* (10 subjects) received IFT (same parameters but a treatment frequency of 80–100 Hz). *Group 5:* (10 subjects) received IFT (same parameters, except no vector and a treatment frequency of 10–20 Hz).	Blood flow was continuously monitored using a laser Doppler probe. Skin temperature was measured throughout the procedure using a skin thermistor probe.	The results demonstrated that a beat frequency of 10–20 Hz produced a significant increase in blood flow. The beat frequency of 10–20 Hz also demonstrated an increase in skin temperature throughout the 30 min duration of the experiment.

Authors	Aim of study	Numbers	Methods	Assessment	Results
Noble et al (2000b)	The purpose of this review was to discuss the current clinical applications of interferential therapy (IFT) with reference to its analgesic potential and possible mechanisms of action.		The authors discuss the various pain theories: gate control, descending pain suppression pathway and physiological block. They then outline the suggested IFT frequencies used to activate the different nerve fibre populations. For example, an IFT frequency of 100 Hz can selectively activate A-beta fibres, utilising the 'pain-gating' system in achieving analgesia. The review looks at the published work on the wide clinical use of IFT. The authors also reviewed IFT studies undertaken for pain relief, incontinence and bone healing.		

Authors	Aim of study	Numbers	Methods	Assessment	Results
Nussbaum et al (1990)	To determine the effects of interferential therapy (IFT) on peripheral blood flow.	55 healthy subjects participated in the study and were assigned to one of three groups.	*Group 1:* (19 subjects) received IFT (carrier frequency 4000 Hz, 4 pole, treatment frequency 0–100 Hz, with vector, at a comfortable intensity for 20 min) applied to the neck region, to include the cervical sympathetic chain and stellate ganglion. *Group 2:* (20 subjects) received IFT (carrier frequency 4000 Hz, 4 pole, treatment frequency 90–100 Hz, with vector, at a comfortable intensity for 20 min) applied to the hand and forearm. *Group 3:* (16 subjects) received IFT (carrier frequency 4000 Hz, 4 pole, treatment frequency 0–150 Hz, with vector, at a comfortable intensity for 20 min) applied either side of the spinal column at T10 to L2 level.	Skin temperature (thermograms) was taken throughout the treatment and post-treatment.	The thermography did not record any skin temperature changes at the areas tested. The authors concluded that IFT did not cause vasodilation.

Authors	Aim of study	Numbers	Methods	Assessment	Results
Pope et al (1995)	To assess the current clinical use of electro-therapeutic modalities in the NHS in England		Interferential therapy (IFT) units (electrodes and suction) were widely owned and frequently used. 207 respondents owned interferential (electrodes) units and only one respondent did not use this modality. Out of 196 respondents, over half (114) used IFT 2–3 times a day and a further 21 respondents used IFT daily. 195 respondents owned interferential (suction) units and 17 respondents did not use this modality. Out of 151 respondents, nearly two-thirds (91) used IFT 2–3 times per day and a further 21 respondents used IFT daily.		
Quirk et al (1985)	To evaluate the effects of interferential therapy (IFT), shortwave diathermy and exercises in the treatment of osteoarthritis (OA) of the knee.	38 patients with OA of the knee were randomly allocated to one of three groups.	*Group 1:* (12 subjects) received IFT (suction electrodes, frequency 0–100 Hz for 10 min and 130 Hz for 5 min) and exercises (straight leg raise (SLR) × 30, twice daily). *Group 2:* (12 subjects) received shortwave diathermy (condenser field method for 20 min) and exercises. *Group 3:* (14 subjects) received exercises only and told to continue to the end of the trial.	Patients were assessed before, on completion of their course of treatment and 3–6 months following completion of their treatment. Range of movement, walking distance, and maximum knee girth were assessed. Pain, using the visual analogue scale (VAS) and function were also	At the end of the treatment, there was a significant improvement in the mean pain scores and overall clinical condition of all three groups.

Authors	Aim of study	Numbers	Methods	Assessment	Results
Shafshak et al (1991)		50 patients with OA of the knee.	50 patients with OA knee pain received bipolar interferential therapy (beat frequency 20–50 Hz and an intensity of a pleasant electric sensation for 10 min). Each patient received daily treatment for 2 weeks (10 sessions). Patients completed the Minnesota Multiphasic Personality Inventory (MMPI) to assess personality traits. Pain relief was assessed by visual analogue scale at the end of treatment and 1 week later. Patients who experienced pain relief of 50% or more were considered responders ($n = 22$). Those who experienced pain relief of 25% or less were considered non-responders ($n = 24$).		No statistical significant difference was found between the two groups on any of the personality traits studied.
Stephenson & Johnson (1995)	To investigate the analgesic effects of interferential therapy (IFT) in healthy subjects.	17 healthy students were assigned to two groups.	Group 1: (7 subjects) received IFT (4 pole, frequency 100 Hz at a 'strong but comfortable' intensity) applied over the anterior aspect of the upper arm to target the median nerve. Group 2: (10 subjects) were a control group and did not receive IFT.	Pain threshold and pain tolerance measurements were taken during six experimental cycles, each lasting 15 min.	Interferential currents significantly increased pain threshold in healthy subjects when compared with a control group.

Authors	Aim of study	Numbers	Methods	Assessment	Results
Vahtera et al (1997)		80 MS patients with lower urinary tract dysfunction were randomly assigned to an active group and a control group.	*The Active Group:* (40 subjects) received interferential therapy (carrier frequency 2000 Hz, treatment frequencies 5–10 Hz, 10–50 Hz, 50 Hz each for 10 min at the maximal tolerable intensity), to the pelvic floor muscles for 6 treatments. This group also received 1–2 sessions of biofeedback for instruction in pelvic floor exercises and advised to continue these 3–5 times a week for 6 months. *The Control Group:* (40 subjects) received no treatment.		The study demonstrated that electrical stimulation with interferential currents activated pelvic floor muscles in MS patients and that such therapy, in combination with regular pelvic floor exercises, improves the symptoms of urinary dysfunction.
Watson (2000)			The author discusses current concepts in electrotherapy, the electrical potential of the cell, high and low energy approaches, frequency and amplitude windows and modalities. The sections on 'interferential' and 'ultrasound' are particularly informative.		

REFERENCES

Adedoyin R A, Olaogun M O B, Fagbeja O O 2002 Effect of interferential current stimulation in management of osteoarthritic knee pain. Physiotherapy 88:493–499

Christie A D, Willoughby G L 1990 The effect of interferential therapy on swelling following open reduction and internal fixation of ankle fractures. Physiotherapy Theory and Practice 6:3–7

Fourie J A, Bowerbank P 1997 Stimulation of bone healing in new fractures of the tibial shaft using interferential currents. Physiotherapy Research International 2:255–268

Hurley D A, Minder P M, McDonough S M et al 2001 Interferential therapy electrode placement technique in acute low back pain: A preliminary investigation. Archives of Physical Medicine and Rehabilitation 82:485–493

Johnson M I 1999 The mystique of interferential currents when used to manage pain. Physiotherapy 85:294–297

Johnson M I, Wilson H 1997 The analgesic effects of different swing patterns of interferential currents on cold-induced pain. Physiotherapy 83:461–467

Lamb S, Mani R 1994 Does interferential therapy affect blood flow? Clinical Rehabilitation 8:213–218

Laycock J, Jerwood D 1993 Does pre-modulated interferential therapy cure genuine stress incontinence? Physiotherapy 79:553–560

Noble J G, Henderson G, Cramp F L et al 2000a The effect of interferential therapy upon cutaneous blood flow in humans. Clinical Physiology 20:2–7

Noble J G, Lowe A S, Walsh D M 2000b Interferential therapy review. Part 1. Mechanism of analgesic action and clinical usage. Physical Therapy Reviews 5:239–245

Nussbaum E, Rush P, Disenhaus L 1990 The effects of interferential therapy on peripheral blood flow. Physiotherapy 76:803–807

Palmer S, Martin D 2002 Interferential current for pain control. In: Kitchen S (ed) Electrotherapy: evidence-based practice, 11th edn. Churchill Livingstone, London, p 287–300

Pope G D, Mockett S P, Wright J P 1995 A survey of electrotherapeutic modalities: ownership and use in the NHS in England. Physiotherapy 81:82–91

Quirk A S, Newman R J, Newman K J 1985 An evaluation of interferential therapy, shortwave diathermy and exercise in the treatment of osteoarthrosis of the knee. Physiotherapy 71:55–57

Robertson V, Ward A, Low J et al 2006 Electrotherapy explained: principles and practice, 4th edn. Elsevier Science, Oxford

Shafshak T S, El-Sheshai A N, Soltan H E 1991 Personality traits in the mechanisms of interferential therapy for osteoarthritic knee pain. Archives of Physical Medicine and Rehabilitation 72:579–581

Stephenson R, Johnson M 1995 The analgesic effects of interferential therapy on cold-induced pain in healthy subjects: A preliminary report. Physiotherapy Theory and Practice 11:89–95

Vahtera T, Viramo-Koskela A L, Ruutiainen J 1997 Pelvic floor rehabilitation is effective in patients with multiple sclerosis. Clinical Rehabilitation 11:211–219

Watson T 2000 The role of electrotherapy in contemporary physiotherapy practice. Manual Therapy 5:132–141

PART 3

BIOSTIMULATION OF TISSUE

Chapter 8 – Pulsed shortwave diathermy   159

Chapter 9 – Ultrasound therapy   185

Chapter 10 – Laser therapy   213

CHAPTER 8

Pulsed shortwave diathermy

PRODUCTION

Pulsed shortwave diathermy (PSWD) is also known as pulsed electromagnetic energy (PEME) or pulsed electromagnetic field (PEMF).

The production of the high frequency current for pulsed shortwave diathermy is exactly the same as for continuous SWD, as it is the same machine. The oscillator circuit induces a current into the patient or resonator circuit. The only difference is the fact that the current is pulsed. As in ultrasound, if the treatment cycle or 'on' time is sufficiently short compared with the 'off' time, then the heating effect is minimal as the tissue is able to disperse the heat generated during 'on' cycles. The mean power delivered to the patient is relatively low, even though the peak power (during the 'on' period) can be quite high.

The mean power delivered needs to be calculated to establish the correct dosage (see Table 8.1). In order to calculate this quickly, it can be attached to the SWD machine as shown at the top left of Figure 8.1.

This modality can be applied using either the condenser/capacitor field method or the inductothermy (cable) method. This can be applied via a drum-type electrode which consists of a flat helical metal coil contained in a plastic casing. This 'circuplode' sets up a magnetic field, producing *eddy currents* in the tissues, which produce heating.

DOSAGE

Acute conditions: use a mean power of <3 Watts. The more acute, the narrower the pulses.
Sub-acute conditions: use a mean power between 3 and 5 Watts. As the condition becomes less acute, use wider pulses.

PRACTICAL ELECTROTHERAPY

Table 8.1 TABLE SHOWING MEAN POWER DELIVERED

Position of intensity controls	1	2	3	4	5	6	7	8	9	10
Maximum pulse power (W)	100	200	300	400	500	600	700	800	900	1000
Pulse repetition frequency										
15 Hz	0.6	1.2	1.8	2.4	3	3.6	4.2	4.8	5.4	6
20 Hz	0.8	1.6	2.4	3.2	4	4.8	5.6	6.4	7.2	8
26 Hz	1.0	2.1	3.2	4.2	5.3	6.4	7.4	8.5	10	11
35 Hz	1.4	2.8	4.2	5.6	7	8.4	9.8	11	13	14
46 Hz	1.9	3.8	5.6	7.5	9.4	11	13	15	17	19
62 Hz	2.5	5	7.5	10	13	15	18	20	23	25
82 Hz	3.3	6.6	10	13	17	20	23	27	30	33
110 Hz	4.4	8.8	13	18	22	27	31	35	40	44
150 Hz	5.9	12	18	24	29	35	41	47	53	59
200 Hz	7.8	16	23	31	39	47	55	63	70	78

Pulsed shortwave diathermy

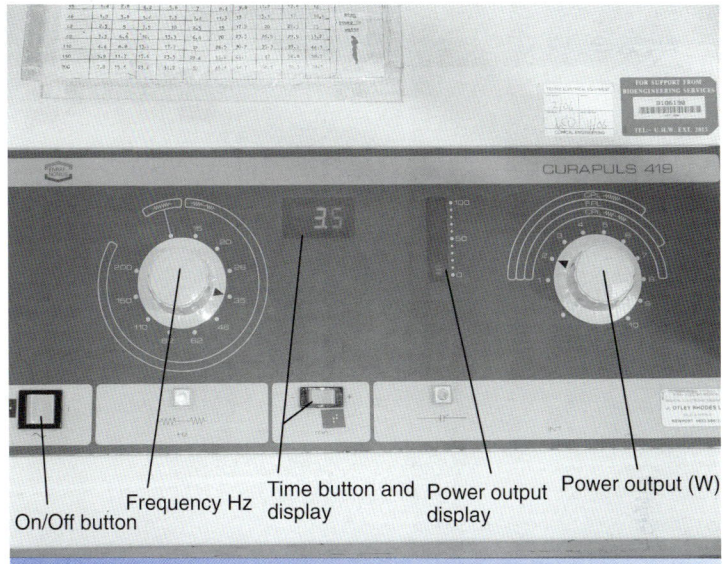

Figure 8.1 Shortwave diathermy/pulsed electromagnetic energy (SWD/PEME) machine and table to calculate the mean dosage.

Chronic conditions: use a power of >5 Watts to achieve a tissue response. At a mean power of >12 Watts, more people can feel some heating effect (Bricknell & Watson 1995, Murray & Kitchen 2000).

Bricknell and Watson (1995) state that a skin sensation test must be carried out on a patient when using PSWD at a mean power in excess of 5 Watts.

APPLICATION

1. Position patient comfortably with the treatment area exposed.
2. Test the machine with your hand or a neon tube (Fig. 8.2).
3. Perform a skin sensation test with the hot and cold test tubes.
4. Dry the skin with a towel.
5. Explain the procedure and re-check for any contraindications to treatment.
6. Mark the position of the joint line.
7. Position the machine as in Figure 8.3, parallel with the upper arm.

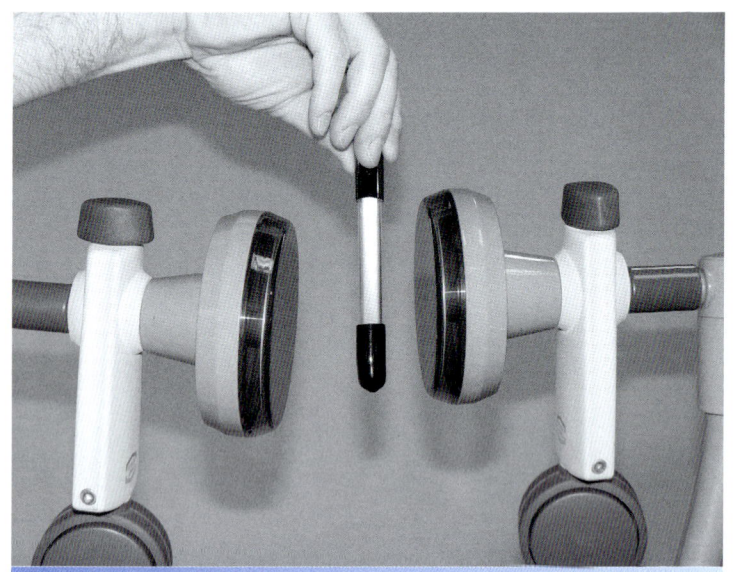

Figure 8.2 Testing the machine with a neon tube. (You could use your hand as in Figure 3.4B.)

8. Position the electrodes parallel and about 2 cm away from the skin. The centre should be in line with the centre of the joint line marked (see Fig. 8.3).
9. Ensure all the cables and leads are a safe distance from the patient.
10. Unlike SWD, this is not a heat treatment (if treating an acute condition). A warmth should not be felt. If even a mild warmth is felt, the treatment should be stopped.
11. Turn the machine on, set the time to 10, 15 or 20 min.
12. Set the pulse frequency and then increase the intensity to produce the desired dosage (given on the table on the machines).
13. Do not leave the area.
14. At the end of the treatment, check the skin for adverse reactions.

ADAPTATIONS

Some machines come with or have a 'circuplode' attachment which can be used to treat one side of a joint or a larger area, such as the back or thigh. These circuplode attachments come in a number of sizes to treat different areas of the body (see Fig. 8.4).

Pulsed shortwave diathermy

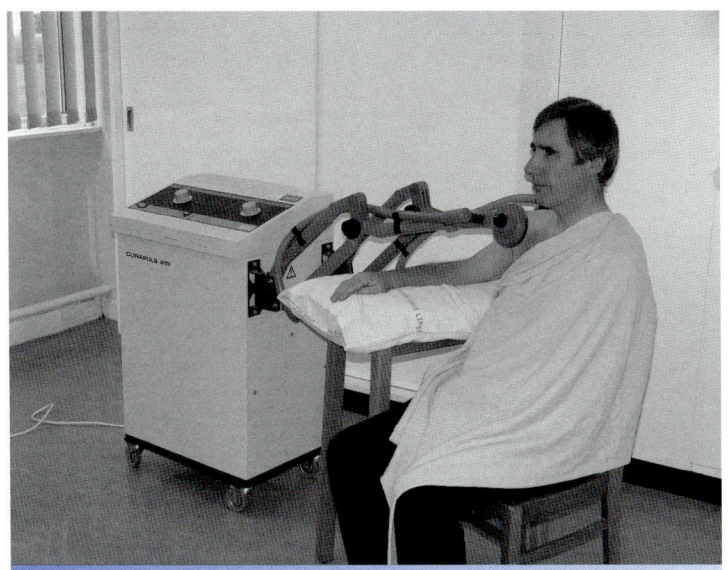

Figure 8.3 Positioning of the machine and electrodes. Pulsed shortwave diathermy (PSWD) to the shoulder using two medium rigid electrodes.

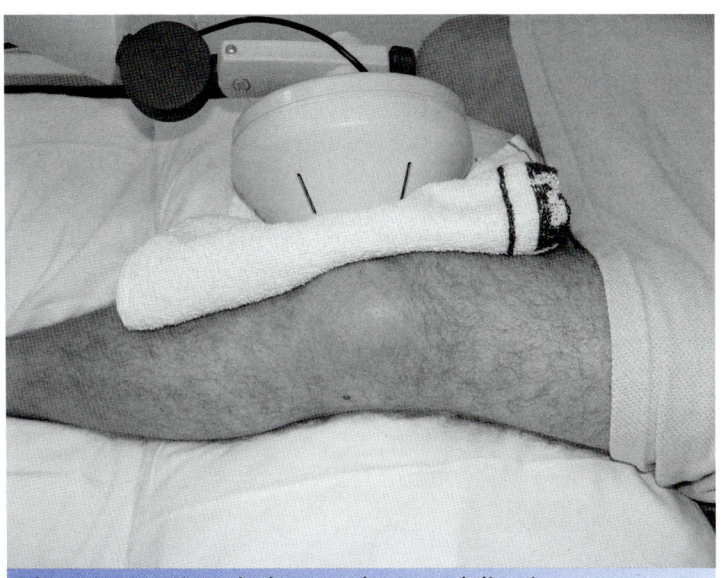

Figure 8.4 'Circuplode' attachment, delivering treatment to the medial aspect of the knee. There is a towel placed between the tissues and the circuplode attachment.

Physiological effects
Increases the number and activity of the cells in the injured region
Reabsorption of haematoma
Reduces swelling and inflammation
Increases rate of fibrin deposition and orientation
Increases collagen deposition and organisation
Increases nerve growth and repair.

Therapeutic uses
Tissue trauma (accident and postoperative)
Recent injuries: sprains, haematomas and acute traumatic synovitis
Acute infection
Bone growth
Wound healing.

Contraindications/precautions
Metal in the area, including implants
Cardiac pacemaker
Synthetic materials
Obese patients
Pregnancy
Implanted slow release hormone capsules
Impaired sensation
Uncooperative or drowsy/unconscious patient
Patient who is unable to sit still.

(See Robertson et al 2006 and Scott 2002.)

Pulsed shortwave diathermy

Notes

166 PRACTICAL ELECTROTHERAPY

Treatment record

Table 8.2 OBSERVATIONAL/REFLECTIVE CHECKLIST

	Observation	Y/N	Comments
Introduction	Did the therapist introduce him/herself?	☐	☐
	Was an explanation of the procedure given?	☐	☐
	Was the explanation clear and succinct?	☐	☐
	Were the possible dangers highlighted?	☐	☐
	Was consent obtained?	☐	☐
Comfort and safety	Was the patient comfortable?	☐	☐
	Was the therapist's posture compromised?	☐	☐
	Was the position safe for both parties?	☐	☐
	Was the modality applied with due care and attention?	☐	☐
Technique	Were the contraindications checked?	☐	☐
	Were the appropriate tests performed prior to treatment?	☐	☐
	Was an explanation of the physiological effects of the technique offered to the patient?	☐	☐
	Was this explanation accurate?	☐	☐
	Was the technique/modality applied correctly?	☐	☐
	Were the correct times and settings used?	☐	☐
	Was the skin checked after the treatment for adverse effects?	☐	☐

Table 8.3 SUMMARY OF STUDIES INVESTIGATING THE EFFECTIVENESS OF PULSED SHORTWAVE DIATHERMY (PSWD)

Authors	Aim of study	Numbers	Methods	Assessment	Results
Ali (2001)	The paper describes a case report of a patient suffering from fibromyalgia, presenting with neck/shoulder/scapular pain, fatigue, disturbed sleep and difficulties in activities of daily living (ADL).		The patient was treated with Maitland spinal mobilisations and McKenzie back extension exercises plus pulsed shortwave diathermy (PSWD) (circuplode electrode, pulse repetition rate 110 Hz, maximum pulse power 400 W, mean power 18 W for 12 min) to right upper trapezius/thoracic spine region for 5 sessions, and ultrasound (3 MHz, intensity of 0.75 W/cm^2 for 4 min to each side of the paravertebral muscles), for 4 sessions.	Pain and fatigue were assessed using the visual analogue scale (VAS). The patient was taking analgesia 4-hourly.	Following nine sessions of physiotherapy, pain and fatigue had reduced, the patient was no longer taking analgesia and the patient was able to sleep through the night. The patient had no difficulties with activities of daily living (ADL).
Barclay et al (1983)	To determine the effectiveness of pulsed electromagnetic energy (PEME), using a Diapulse unit, in the treatment of various hand injuries.	60 patients with an injury to the hand or thumb were randomly assigned to a treatment and a control group.	The Treatment Group: received routine hand treatment plus PEME to the hand, using a Diapulse unit (frequency 27.12 MHz, 975 W in short bursts of 65 μs followed by a rest period of 1600 μs, for 30 min), twice daily until discharge. The Control Group: received routine hand treatment.	Measurements were taken of swelling (tape measure), disability (measurement of finger flexion using a tape measure) and pain (5-point scale). Measurements were taken on the 1st day of treatment and the 3rd, 5th and 7th days.	Those patients receiving PEME demonstrated a significant reduction in swelling ($p < 0.001$), which also had a marked effect on function and pain.

Authors	Aim of study	Numbers	Methods	Assessment	Results
Bricknell & Watson (1995)	To establish the power required to give a thermal effect in the tissues when using pulsed shortwave diathermy (PSWD).	40 healthy students were randomly allocated to an experimental group and a control group.	*The Experimental Group:* (32 subjects) received PSWD using a circuplode electrode (pulse duration 400 μs, pulse repetition rate 400 Hz, mean power of 1.6 W) to the mid-point of the thigh. The PSWD was applied continuously for 30 min, the mean power being increased by 0.8 W every 30 s until a definite thermal sensation was achieved. *The Control Group:* (8 subjects) had an identical procedure, except the mean power was kept at 0.01 W, pulse duration 65 μs, pulse repetition rate 26 Hz for 15 min.	Skin temperature was measured using a digital thermometer and temperature probe. This was measured initially and after the subjects had expressed a 'definite' identification of warmth.	Their findings suggest that a significant relationship exists between the definite thermal perception and skin temperature post-treatment ($p < 0.001$) and demonstrated a significant difference between initial and post-treatment temperatures in the experimental group ($p < 0.001$).
Buzzard et al (2003)	To compare ice therapy using cryocuff with pulsed shortwave diathermy (PSWD), for the reduction of oedema following calcaneal fractures.	20 patients with acute calcaneal fractures were randomly assigned to receive one of two interventions.	Nine patients received PSWD (pulse frequency 26 Hz, pulse duration 200 μs, intensity of 35 W for 15 min), twice daily for 5 days. 11 patients received the ice therapy (cryocuff) for 20 min, 6 times a day for 5 days.	Swelling around the ankle and foot was measured using a tape measure. Range of movement (dorsiflexion, plantarflexion, inversion and eversion) was measured using a goniometer.	All 20 subjects gained a significant increase in all ankle movements ($p = 0.007$). There was no notable reduction in swelling in either group. PSWD was not demonstrated to be substantially better in oedema reduction following calcaneal fractures.

Authors	Aim of study	Numbers	Methods	Assessment	Results
Callaghan et al (2000)	To employ established radioleuco-scintigraphy techniques to evaluate objectively the effect of pulsed shortwave diathermy (PSWD) on the inflammatory component of the osteoarthritic (OA) knee.	27 patients with OA knees were randomly allocated to three groups.	Group 1: (9 subjects) received PSWD (pulse duration 200 μs, pulse frequency 400 Hz, output of 10 W for 20 min) to the affected knee. Group 2: (9 subjects) received PSWD (pulse duration 400 μs, pulse frequency 400 Hz, output of 20 W for 20 min) to the affected knee. Group 3: (9 subjects) received sham PSWD for 20 min and acted as a control.	The measurements assessed were range of movement, pain, muscle strength, timed walk and radioleuco-scintigraphy.	The results showed there were no significant differences between the groups in the pre- and post-treatment percentage change for radioleucoscintigraphy ($p > 0.05$) or functional and subject measures ($p > 0.05$). The authors concluded that this method of treatment had little or no anti-inflammatory effect on this condition.
Dziedzic et al (2005)	To investigate whether manual therapy (with advice and exercises) or pulsed shortwave diathermy (PSWD; with advice and exercises) was better than advice	350 patients with non-specific neck disorders were randomly assigned to three groups.	Group 1: (115 subjects) were given advice and exercises during a 20-min session. Group 2: (114 subjects) were given advice and exercises with the addition of manual therapy during a 20-min session. Group 3: (121 subjects) were given advice and exercises with the	The outcome measures used were the Northwick Park Neck Pain Questionnaire and the participants' global assessment of change compared with baseline.	The authors concluded that the addition of manual therapy and PSWD to advice and exercises did not provide any further benefit in the treatment of neck disorders.

Authors	Aim of study	Numbers	Methods	Assessment	Results
	and exercise alone in the treatment of non-specific neck disorders.		addition of PSWD (no indication of how PSWD was delivered or what parameters were used) during a 20-min session. All participants received eight sessions.		
Grant et al (1989)	To determine the effectiveness of ultrasound and pulsed electromagnetic energy (PEME) treatment for perineal trauma.	414 patients with perineal trauma were randomly allocated to one of four groups.	*Group 1*: (140 subjects) received active ultrasound (frequency of 3 MHz, pulsed 1:4, intensity of 0.5 W/cm² for 2 min) to each area of trauma. *Group 2*: (135 subjects) received active PEME (pulse frequency of 100 Hz, pulse width of 65 μs for 10 min) to the area of trauma. *Groups 3 and 4*: (139 subjects) received 'sham' ultrasound or PEME.	Patients were assessed for pain using the visual analogue scale (VAS), extent of oedema, bruising and haemorrhoids and any analgesia over the course of the treatment. A further assessment was undertaken after 10 days and then by questionnaire 3 months postpartum.	At the post-treatment assessment 91% of the participants felt the treatment had made them better. There were no clear differences between the groups in outcome either immediately after treatment, or 10 days or 3 months postpartum.

Authors	Aim of study	Numbers	Methods	Assessment	Results
Gray et al (1995)	To evaluate and compare the effects of four different electrotherapeutic modalities, namely shortwave diathermy, megapulse (pulsed shortwave diathermy), ultrasound and laser therapy on patients with temporomandibular pain dysfunction (TMPDS).	139 patients with TMPDS were randomly allocated into five groups.	*Group 1:* (27 subjects) received shortwave diathermy at a mild setting for 10 min. *Group 2:* (27 subjects) received megapulse (pulsed shortwave) (pulse frequency 100 Hz, pulse duration 60 µs) for 20 min. *Group 3:* (30 subjects) received ultrasound (3 MHz, pulsed 2:1, intensity of 0.25 W/cm² for 2 min. *Group 4:* (29 subjects) received laser therapy (wavelength 904 nm, dosage of 4 J/cm²) for 3 min. *Group 5:* (26 subjects) received placebo treatment with one of the above modalities. All participants received treatment 3 times a week for 4 weeks.	Assessment of improvement was made objectively on the basis of a total symptom profile. Those symptoms recorded pre- and post-treatment were muscle tenderness, joint sounds and joint tenderness on direct palpation. Range of movement (ROM) was measured and the subjective improvement was recorded on the basis of the patients' report on their overall state (worse, unchanged, variable, much better or cured).	At the time of the first review, 7 days after the completion of treatment, there was no significant difference in the success rate between any of the treatment groups or between the treated and placebo groups. At the final review, at 3 months, a definite and significant difference between the treated and placebo groups had emerged.

Authors	Aim of study	Numbers	Methods	Assessment	Results
Hill et al (2002)	To investigate the hypothesis that pulsed shortwave diathermy (PSWD) directly accelerates fibroblast cell proliferation rates *in vitro* and to establish the influences of different dosage variables.		In a controlled laboratory setting, four single-blind trials were completed to investigate the influences of PSWD irradiation rates *in vitro* on fibroblast and chondrocyte cell division rates. To assess the effect of PSWD on fibroblast proliferation, PSWD (peak pulse power 150 W, frequency 800 Hz, pulse width 400 μs, mean power of 48 W) was placed 2 cm from a microtiter plate and applied for 10 min, twice daily.	The outcome measure for each experiment was optical density (a proxy measure of cell numbers). Optical density was ascertained spectrophotometrically in a plate reader at a known wavelength of 600 nm. These cells were human adult dermal fibroblasts and chondrocytes, plated at known concentrations and incubated for 5 days.	The optical density was compared with that of a control group not exposed to PSWD. The effect of PSWD proved significant ($p < 0.001$). The assessment of the relationship between mean power dosage and fibroblast proliferation, estimated the optimal optical density at the PSWD dosage corresponding to 13.8 W. At a constant dosage of 6 W, chondrocyte proliferation varied significantly with treatment duration ($p < 0.001$). All treatment groups had significantly better optical densities than the control group

Authors	Aim of study	Numbers	Methods	Assessment	Results
					($p < 0.015$). The authors concluded that PSWD had a significant influence on fibroblast and chondrocyte proliferation in the laboratory setting.
Kitchen & Partridge (1992)	This is an extensive paper discussing the physical effects of continuous and pulsed shortwave diathermy and their physiological effects, with regard to the thermal and athermal mechanisms. The efficacy of both continuous and pulsed shortwave diathermy is examined through the use of both experimental models (animal studies) and clinical trials. Experimental studies have been undertaken on soft tissues and joints, whereas clinical trials have been undertaken on soft tissues, joint studies and pain relief. Hazards to shortwave diathermy have been identified.				
Klaber Moffett et al (1996)	To investigate the effectiveness of pulsed shortwave diathermy (PSWD) in the relief of pain on osteoarthritis (OA) of the hip and knee.	75 patients with OA of the hip or knee were randomly allocated to three groups.	Group 1: (26 subjects) received PSWDS (circuplode, pulse frequency 82 Hz, pulse duration 400 µs, maximum pulse power 77 W, mean power 23 W), for 15 min, 3 times weekly for 3 weeks, to the centre of the joint. Group 2: (22 subjects) received 'sham' PSWD, set-up as above. Group 3: (27 subjects) acted as a control group and received no treatment.	Patients were assessed using a pain diary (using a numerical rating scale of 0–100), a subjective pain report (numerical rating scale of 0–100), a General Health Questionnaire and Activities of Daily Living.	Patients in the placebo group reported more benefit from treatment than those in the active treatment group. The authors conclude that active PSWD, as administered in this study, was not specifically beneficial for this patient population.

Authors	Aim of study	Numbers	Methods	Assessment	Results
Laufer et al (2005)	To examine whether there were any differences between pulsed shortwave diathermy (PSWD), delivered at an intensity sufficient to induce a thermal sensation or at an athermal sensation, and a placebo treatment in terms of their effect on pain, stiffness and functional ability of patients with osteoarthritic (OA) knees.	103 patients with OA of the knee were sequentially allocated to three groups.	*Group 1:* (32 subjects) received high-intensity PSWD (circuplode, pulse duration 300 μs, pulse frequency of 300 Hz, peak power 200 W, mean power 18 W), to the anterior aspect of the knee. *Group 2:* (38 subjects) received low-intensity PSWD (circuplode, pulse duration 82 μs, pulse frequency 110 Hz, peak power 200 W, mean power 1.8 W), to the knee. *Group 3:* (33 subjects) received 'sham' shortwave diathermy (SWD) to the knee. All participants received treatment for 20 min, 3 times a week for 3 weeks.	Patients were assessed pre-test, post-test and 12 weeks following the last treatment. Patients were assessed using the WOMAC Osteoarthritis Index (assessing pain, stiffness and functional ability), the Timed-Get-Up and-Go test, timed stair-climbing, timed stair-descending and 3-min walk.	The results of the present study demonstrated no differences between the effects of PSWD and a SWD placebo treatment on the self-reported measures of pain, stiffness and functional activity (WOMAC) or on objective measures of functional performance. The authors conclude that the findings of this study seriously question the efficacy of PSWD for the treatment of OA.

Authors	Aim of study	Numbers	Methods	Assessment	Results
Low (1995)	This paper discusses the mechanisms by which pulsed shortwave diathermy (PSWD) might be therapeutically effective. The most simple mechanism is that PSWD simply 'stirs' ions, molecules, membranes and metabolic activity of cells; increasing the overall rates of phagocytosis, transport across membranes, enzymic activity, etc. This leads to the acceleration of inflammatory and healing processes and resolution of injury. Another mechanism proposed is that an electromagnetic field is able to alter the cell membrane potential, re-polarising the cell. A further mechanism is that 'high or low intensity electromagnetic energy delivered at whatever frequency or pulse length will ultimately end as heat whatever other energy conversions may also occur'. The author discusses nine clinical trials using PSWD to treat acute tissue injuries. He analyses the treatment parameters (pulse frequency, pulse width, peak power, mean power, energy applied per 24 h) used in these trials.				
Murray & Kitchen (2000)	The purpose of the study was to determine the pulse repetition rate (PRR) required to generate a 'possible' and 'definite' thermal sensation when pulsed shortwave diathermy (PSWD) was applied to the mid-point of the thigh.	30 healthy students were randomly divided into a treatment and a placebo group.	The authors tested a range of PRRs from 26 Hz to 400 Hz in 10 increments, maintaining a constant pulse duration of 400 μs and peak power of 190 W.	Skin temperature of the thigh was measured using a thermistor and probe.	Their findings suggest that a significant relationship existed between skin temperature and post-treatment and PRR at the 'possible' ($p < 0.001$) and 'definite' ($p < 0.001$) thermal perception.

Authors	Aim of study	Numbers	Methods	Assessment	Results
Peres et al (2002)	To compare the effects of combining pulsed shortwave diathermy (PSWD), with or without ice, with prolonged long-duration calf stretching on (1) daily changes in flexibility, (2) day-to-day changes in flexibility and (3) retention of flexibility 6 days after cessation of treatment.	44 healthy students were randomly assigned to one of five groups.	*Group 1:* (8 subjects) acted as a control and received stretching to the triceps surae for 10 min. *Group 2:* (8 subjects) acted as a second control and were measured before and at the end of the study. *Group 3:* (11 subjects) received stretching to the triceps surae for 10 min. *Group 4:* (8 subjects) received heat (PSWD, circuplode, pulse frequency of 800 Hz, pulse duration 400 µs, interburst intervals of 800 µs, peak power of 150 W, mean power of 48 W) applied for 20 min and stretching. *Group 5:* (9 subjects) received heat (PSWD as above), stretching and ice (ice pack) for 5 min. All participants received treatment 14 times in 3 weeks.	Ankle dorsiflexion was measured using a digital inclinometer before and after treatment and 6 days after the last treatment.	The results suggested that vigorous deep heating (PSWD), combined with prolonged stretching, was more effective than prolonged stretching alone in increasing flexibility throughout the 3 weeks. The authors conclude that PSWD applied before stretching is a safe and effective protocol for increasing tissue extensibility.

Authors	Aim of study	Numbers	Methods	Assessment	Results
Pope et al (1995)	To assess the current clinical use of electrotherapeutic modalities in the NHS in England.		Pulsed shortwave diathermy (PSWD) and shortwave diathermy (SWD) units were widely owned and frequently used. 209 respondents owned PSWD units and only six respondents did not use this modality. Out of 190 respondents, over two-thirds (132) used PSWD 2–3 times a day and a further 20 respondents used PSWD daily. 196 respondents owned SWD units and 68 respondents did not use this modality. Out of 113 respondents, only 22 used SWD 2–3 times/day and a further 12 respondents used SWD daily.		

Authors	Aim of study	Numbers	Methods	Assessment	Results
Seaborne et al (1996)	To evaluate the effectiveness of pulsed electromagnetic energy (PEME) in the treatment of pressure sores, using four different treatment protocols.	20 elderly patients with pressure sores in the trochanteric or sacral regions were randomly allocated to one of four treatment protocols.	In this study an ABAB repeated measures design was used. It permits controlled testing without a separate control group, each patient serving as their own control. *Group 1*: received PEME (circuplode, pulse duration 400 μs, pulse rate frequency 20 Hz, peak pulse power of 700 W, mean pulse power 5.6 W), applied over the sore for 20 min, twice daily. *Group 2*: received PEME (circuplode, pulse duration 400 μs, pulse rate frequency 110 Hz, peak pulse power of 700 W, mean pulse power 30.8 W), applied over the sore for 20 min, twice daily. *Group 3*: received PEME (2 rigid electrodes, same parameters as Group 1, delivering a mean power of 5.6 W), applied either side of the sore. *Group 4*: received PEME (two rigid electrodes, same parameters as Group 2, delivered at a mean power of 30.8 W), applied either side of the sore. All participants received a routine nursing procedure and 20 treatments in total.	The pressure sore area was measured by tracing the outline on sterile transparent wrap. These measurements were taken at the beginning of each week of the study and immediately following the final treatment (five measures in all).	The findings of this study suggest that PEME, using the electric and magnetic fields, at low power densities, can be an effective treatment for pressure sores.

Authors	Aim of study	Numbers	Methods	Assessment	Results
Shields et al (2002)	To establish the current clinical and safety practices during CSWD and PSWD application in Ireland.	83 questionnaires.	Questionnaires were sent to Irish-based physiotherapy departments using SWD. (There was a 75% return.)	PSWD was the preferred mode. CSWD was rated effective for treating chronic osteoarthritis, polyarthritis, non-specific arthrosis, haematomas, acute arthritis, sinusitis and rheumatoid arthritis. There were questions concerning safety practices.	
Shields et al (2004)	To investigate the documented evidence for the contraindications to shortwave diathermy (SWD) and to determine the level of agreement among senior physiotherapists.	116 questionnaires were distributed to Irish physiotherapists.	Irish physiotherapists were asked to categorise 35 symptoms or conditions as either 'always', 'sometimes', or 'never' contraindicated, or 'don't know' whether contraindicated for both continuous and pulsed shortwave diathermy.		There was a 75% response rate. There was over 90% agreement found among respondents for traditional contraindications to both continuous shortwave diathermy (metal implants, pacemakers, malignancy, tuberculous joints, over the eyes) and pulsed shortwave diathermy (malignancy and pacemakers). The authors conclude that there is an overall lack of research-based evidence regarding most contraindications to treatment.

Authors	Aim of study	Numbers	Methods	Assessment	Results
Shields et al (2005)	To investigate how physiotherapists perceive the risk exposure to stray radiofrequency radiation (electromagnetic fields) in the physiotherapy department, in particular the use of shortwave diathermy.	225 questionnaires were sent to physiotherapists working in hospital-based physiotherapy departments.	The questionnaire consisted of four sections. Section 1 consisted of background data questions. Section 2 required respondents to rate their perception of risk for 23 items. Section 3 asked respondents to rate the level of health consequences they perceived would occur from exposure to 22 of the 23 risk items. In section 4, respondents were asked how often they would be able to protect themselves from exposure to 15 risks. Microsoft Access and SPSS statistical packages were used for data analysis.	Of the 225 questionnaires delivered, 203 were completed (90.2%). Respondents were found to perceive exposure to electromagnetic fields (EMFs) as low risk. The respondents also felt they could often protect themselves from the risk of stray EMFs. The authors concluded that respondents were complacent about the dangers involved and therefore there were few safety measures.	
van Nguyen & Marks (2002)	To examine the rationale for, and the potential efficacy of applying pulsed electromagnetic fields (PEMFs) for reducing joint pain and other related symptoms of osteoarthritis (OA).		This paper is a review of laboratory and clinical research studies that have investigated the effects of pulsed electromagnetic fields for the treatment of OA. The authors undertook a systematic search of the literature. This revealed six studies, non-randomised comparative and randomised controlled trials (RCTs), which were reviewed by the authors.		The authors conclude by stating that PEMFs can promote tissue healing and relieve pain and inflammation. The literature suggests PEMF therapy may prove beneficial in the treatment of painful osteoarthritis.

REFERENCES

Ali H M 2001 Fibromyalgia: case report. Physiotherapy 87:140–145

Barclay V, Collier R J, Jones A 1983 Treatment of various hand injuries by pulsed electromagnetic energy (Diapulse). Physiotherapy 69:186–188

Bricknell A T, Watson T 1995 The thermal effects of pulsed shortwave diathermy. British Journal of Therapy and Rehabilitation 2:430–434

Buzzard B M, Pratt R K, Briggs P J et al 2003 Is pulsed shortwave diathermy better than ice therapy for the reduction of oedema following calcaneal fractures? Physiotherapy 89:734–742

Callaghan M J, Whittaker P A, Grimes S et al 2000 An evaluation of pulsed shortwave on knee osteoarthritis using radioleucoscintigraphy: a randomised, double blind, controlled trial. Joint Bone Spine 72:150–155

Dziedzic K, Hill J, Lewis M et al 2005 Effectiveness of manual therapy or pulsed shortwave diathermy in addition to advice and exercise for neck disorders: a pragmatic randomized controlled trial in physical therapy clinics. Arthritis and Rheumatism 53:214–222

Grant A, Sleep J, McIntosh J, Ashurst H 1989 Ultrasound and pulsed electromagnetic energy treatment for perineal trauma. A randomised placebo-controlled trial. British Journal of Obstetrics and Gynaecology 96:434–439

Gray R J M, Hall C A, Quayle A A et al 1995 Temporomandibular pain dysfunction; can electrotherapy help? Physiotherapy 81:47–51

Hill J, Lewis M, Mills P et al 2002 Pulsed short-wave diathermy effects on human fibroblast proliferation. Archives of Physical Medicine and Rehabilitation 83:832–836

Kitchen S, Partridge C 1992 Review of shortwave diathermy continuous and pulsed patterns. Physiotherapy 78:243–252

Klaber Moffett J A, Richardson P H, Frost H et al 1996 A placebo controlled double blind trial to evaluate the effectiveness of pulsed short wave therapy for osteoarthritic hip and knee pain. Pain 67:121–127

Laufer Y, Zilberman R, Porat R et al 2005 Effect of pulsed short-wave diathermy on pain and function of subjects with osteoarthritis of the knee: a placebo-controlled double-blind clinical trial. Clinical Rehabilitation 19:255–263

Low J 1995 Dosage of some pulsed shortwave clinical trials. Physiotherapy 81:611–616

Murray C C, Kitchen S 2000 Effect of pulsed repetition rate on the perception of thermal sensation with pulsed shortwave diathermy. Physiotherapy Research International 5:73–84

Peres S E, Draper D O, Knight K L et al 2002 Pulsed shortwave diathermy and prolonged long-duration stretching increases dorsiflexion range of motion more than identical stretching without diathermy. Journal of Athletic Training 37:43–50

Pope G D, Mockett S P, Wright J P 1995 A survey of electrotherapy modalities: ownership and use in the NHS in England. Physiotherapy 81:82–91

Robertson V, Ward A, Low J et al 2006 Electrotherapy explained: principles and practice, 4th edn. Elsevier Science, Oxford

Scott S 2002 Diathermy. In: Kitchen S (ed) Electrotherapy: evidence-based practice, 11th edn. Churchill Livingstone, London, p 145–170

Seaborne D, Quirion-DeGirardi C, Rousseau M et al 1996 The treatment of pressure sores using pulsed electromagnetic energy (PEME). Physiotherapy Canada Spring 48:131–137

Shields N, Gormley J, O'Hare N 2002 Contraindications to continuous and pulsed short-wave diathermy. Physical Therapy Review 7:133–143

Shields N, Gormley J, O'Hare N 2004 Contraindications to short wave diathermy: Survey of Irish physiotherapists. Physiotherapy 90:42–53

Shields N, Gormley J, O'Hare N 2005 Physiotherapist's perception of risk from electromagnetic fields. Advances in Physiotherapy 7:170–175

van Nguyen J P, Marks R 2002 Pulsed electromagnetic fields for treating osteoarthritis. Physiotherapy 88:458–470

CHAPTER 9

Ultrasound therapy

SOUND WAVES

Ultrasound (U/S), as the name suggests, is a treatment which utilises sound waves to produce physiological effects. Ultrasound refers to mechanical vibration, essentially the same as sound waves, but at a higher frequency (Robertson et al 2006).

Sound waves are a series of mechanical compressions and rarefactions in the direction of travel of the wave. They are longitudinal waves (Robertson et al 2006).

Sound is produced by a moving surface, e.g. the diaphragm in a speaker. As the surface moves forwards, it *compresses* the molecules immediately in front. These molecules in turn push forwards against their neighbours in an attempt to restore their former arrangement. These in turn push *their* neighbours, etc. The compression wave moves away from the source.

If the surface now moves in the opposite direction, the density of the molecules is reduced next to it (an area of *rarefaction*) and so the molecules move in to fill the space. This in turn leaves a low density region, which is immediately filled in by more molecules, so the rarefaction moves away from the source. It is therefore only the form of the sound wave which moves forward; the actual particles vibrate back and forth, around a stationary point.

THE PRODUCTION OF ULTRASOUND

Ultrasound is generated using a *piezoelectric* transducer (head). The quartz crystal in the transducer has the property to change shape when a current is applied across it. Therefore, if an alternating voltage is applied across the crystal it will alternately get thicker and thinner.

The front plate of the transducer is fused to the crystal and therefore as the crystal gets thicker and thinner, the front plate will move forwards and backwards. This movement of the plate will cause regions of *compression* and *rarefaction* in the tissues to which they have been applied (forming an ultrasound wave, see Fig. 9.1).

Therapeutic ultrasound utilises the 'near field' and the wave pattern is irregular. To cancel out these 'irregularities', the treatment head must be continuously moved during the treatment.

Sound waves obey the laws of reflection. Air will not transmit U/S waves. There will be some reflection at each interface that the U/S beam encounters. This gives rise to the term *acoustic impedance*, which is the ratio between the reflected and transmitted U/S at the interface. When the *acoustic impedance* is low, transmission is high.

Once the U/S beam has left the transducer, its intensity is gradually reduced (attenuation). This is primarily due to *absorption* and *scatter*. U/S is *absorbed* in the tissues and converted to heat (thermal effects). *Scatter* occurs when the U/S beam is deflected from its pathway. The U/S beam is therefore reduced in intensity the deeper it passes.

The 'half value distance' is the depth of soft tissue that reduces the U/S beam to half its surface intensity. The half value distance varies from 1 MHz to 3 MHz and is 4 cm and 2.5 cm, respectively (Robertson et al 2006, Young 2002).

EQUIPMENT

Ultrasound machine (see Fig. 9.2)
Hot and cold test tubes for discrimination testing (continuous U/S use)
Transmission gel
Bowl of water and paper towels (not shown).

APPLICATION

1. Test the machine using a bowl of water.
2. Position the patient comfortably and expose the area to be treated.
3. Re-check for any contraindications.
4. Identify the structure/area to be treated and mark.
5. Apply a small amount of gel (see Fig. 9.3).
6. Put the U/S head against the area to be treated and turn on the machine.

Ultrasound therapy

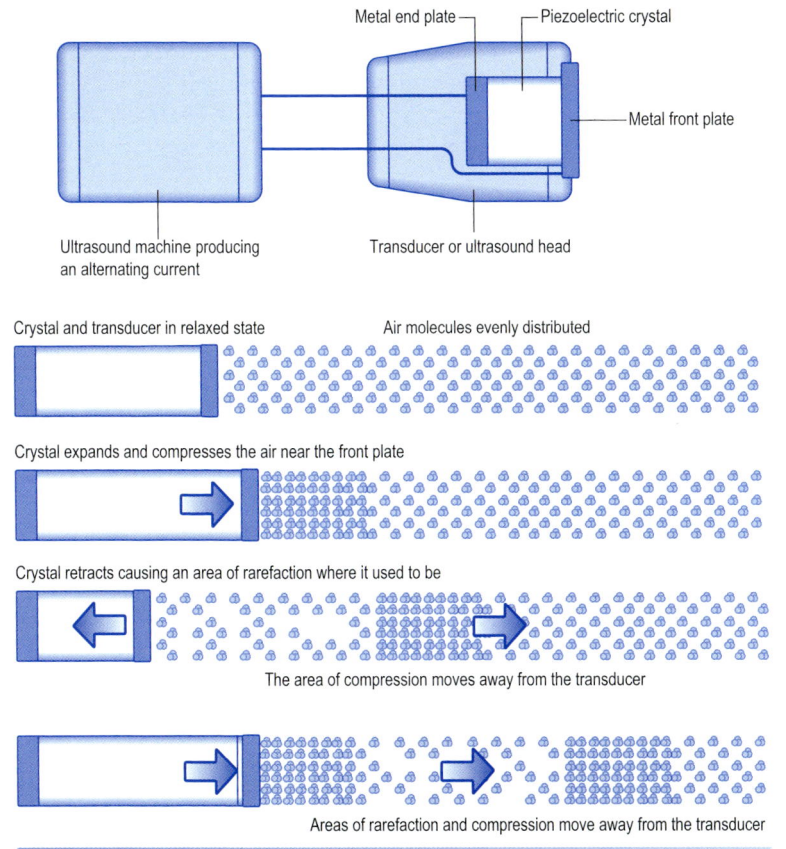

Figure 9.1 Diagram of an ultrasound (U/S) machine and production of sound waves.

Labels: Metal end plate; Piezoelectric crystal; Metal front plate; Ultrasound machine producing an alternating current; Transducer or ultrasound head; Crystal and transducer in relaxed state; Air molecules evenly distributed; Crystal expands and compresses the air near the front plate; Crystal retracts causing an area of rarefaction where it used to be; The area of compression moves away from the transducer; Areas of rarefaction and compression move away from the transducer.

7. Keep the ultrasound head moving when the machine is turned on. Use small slow circles to cover the structure/area.
8. Set the mode of treatment (continuous or pulsed).
9. Set the time (usually 1 min per 1 cm^2).
10. Set the intensity and start the treatment.
11. Ensure the head remains in contact with the skin and that it is kept in motion throughout the treatment.
12. Once treatment time expires, remove the gel and check the area for any adverse affects.

188 PRACTICAL ELECTROTHERAPY

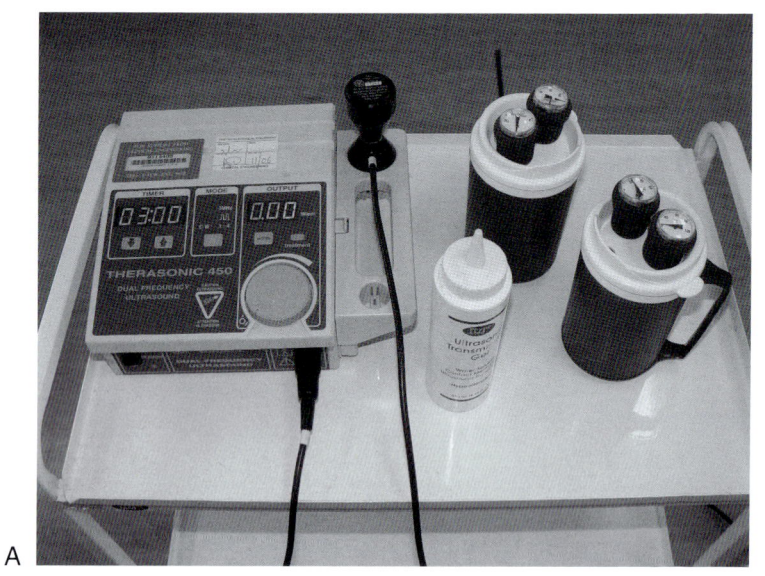

Figure 9.2 (A) Equipment required for U/S treatment. (B) Settings.

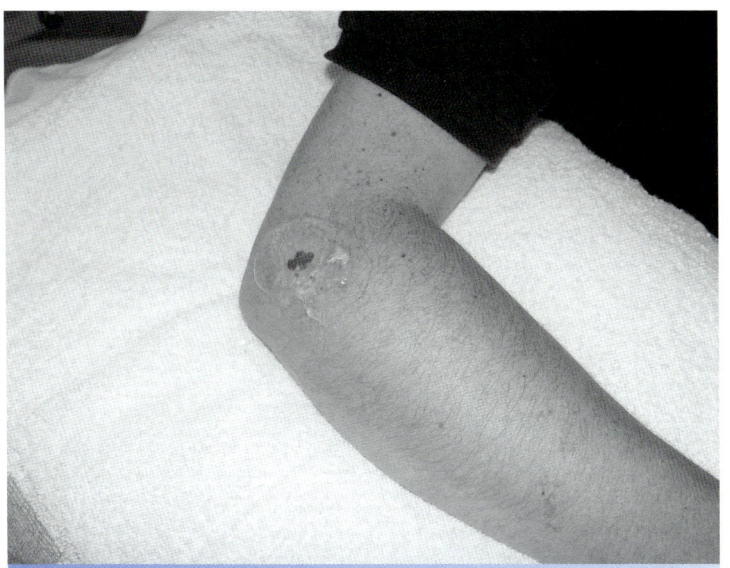

Figure 9.3 Ultrasound gel and mark visible on the lateral epicondyle of the humerus.

ADAPTATIONS
Physiological effects
There are two main effects of ultrasound, thermal and non-thermal, according to whether treatment mode is continuous or pulsed.

Thermal effects
- Kinetic energy from the sound waves is converted to heat via friction.
- The effects of heating are
  - Decreased pain perception
  - Decreased fluid viscosity
  - Increased tissue extensibility above 40°C
  - Increased metabolic rate
  - Increased blood flow; assists in reducing swelling.

Non-thermal effects
- Acoustic streaming
- Cavitation (bubble formation)
- Microstreaming.

All three of these effects can cause membrane distortion and increase permeability, improve transfer of nutrients and

190 PRACTICAL ELECTROTHERAPY

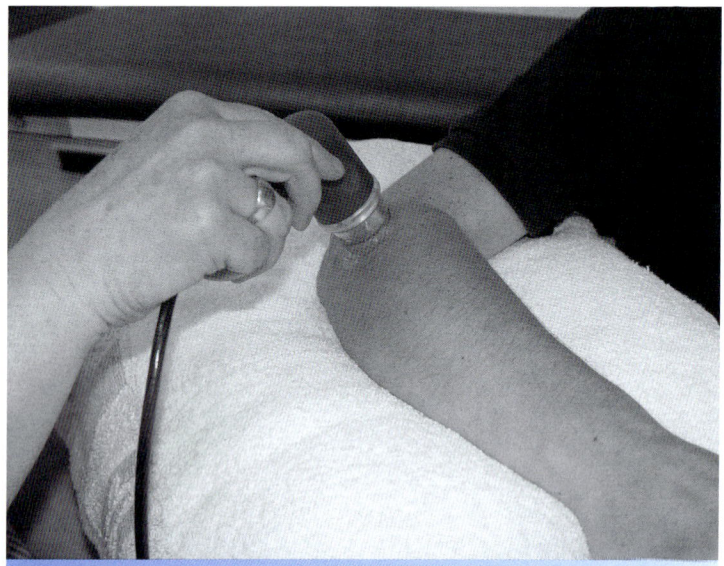

Figure 9.4 U/S applied to the common extensor origin. *Note* the treatment head is at 90° to the tissue. The head should be moved in a slow, circular motion.

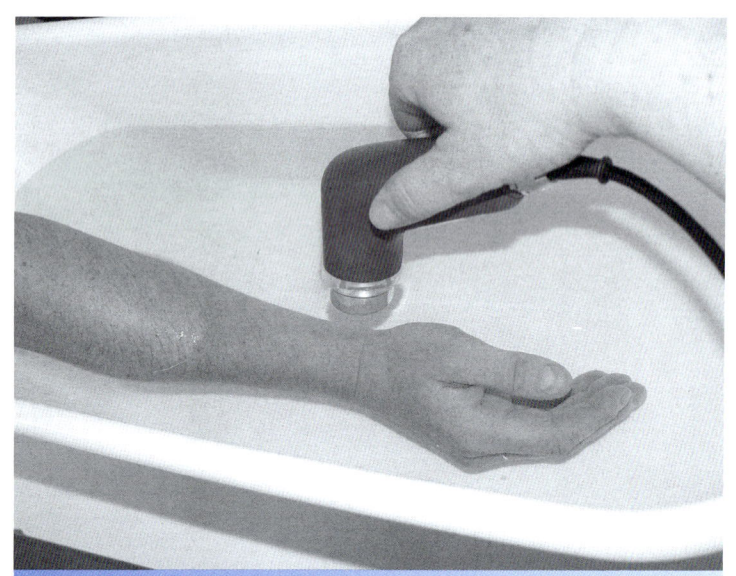

Figure 9.5 U/S can be applied under water if the area is uneven. The head does not touch the skin but remains 1 cm away from it. The head should be 90° to the tissues, moving in a slow, circular motion.

metabolites and facilitate the inflammatory and proliferation phases of healing.

Contraindications
Venous thrombosis
Acute sepsis
Tumours
Deep X-ray therapy
Local infections
Vascular insufficiency
Active TB
Metal implants
Pacemakers
Central nervous tissue
Uncontrolled bleeding or anticoagulant therapy
Over the eyes, reproductive organs or a pregnant uterus.

Precautions
Acute inflammation
Epiphyseal growth plates
Decreased sensation
Standing waves: this is where the reflected wave is superimposed on the incident wave. This can lead to damaged tissue and is prevented by keeping the head moving, taking care over bony prominences and also by using pulsed mode.

(See Robertson et al 2006 and Young 2002.)

Notes

Ultrasound therapy 193

Treatment record

Table 9.1 *OBSERVATIONAL/REFLECTIVE CHECKLIST*

	Observation	Y/N	Comments
Introduction	Did the therapist introduce him/herself?	☐	☐
	Was an explanation of the procedure given?	☐	☐
	Was the explanation clear and succinct?	☐	☐
	Were the possible dangers highlighted?	☐	☐
	Was consent obtained?	☐	☐
Comfort and safety	Was the patient comfortable?	☐	☐
	Was the therapist's posture compromised?	☐	☐
	Was the position safe for both parties?	☐	☐
	Was the modality applied with due care and attention?	☐	☐
Technique	Were the contraindications checked?	☐	☐
	Were the appropriate tests performed prior to treatment?	☐	☐
	Was an explanation of the physiological effects of the technique offered to the patient?	☐	☐
	Was this explanation accurate?	☐	☐
	Was the technique/modality applied correctly?	☐	☐
	Were the correct times and settings used?	☐	☐
	Was the skin checked after the treatment for adverse effects?	☐	☐

Ultrasound therapy

Table 9.2 SUMMARY OF STUDIES INVESTIGATING THE EFFECTIVENESS OF ULTRASOUND THERAPY (U/S)

Authors	Aim of study	Numbers	Methods	Assessment	Results
Baker et al (2001)			The purpose of the review was to examine the literature regarding the biophysical effects (the thermal and non-thermal effects) of therapeutic ultrasound to determine whether these may be considered sufficient to provide a biological rationale for the use of insonation for the treatment of people with pain and soft tissue injury.		The authors conclude that the review indicates that the biophysical effects of ultrasound are unlikely to be beneficial due to there being insufficient evidence.
Binder et al (1985)	To assess the effectiveness of ultrasound in the treatment of lateral epicondylitis (tennis elbow).	76 patients with lateral epicondylitis were randomly assigned to a treatment group or placebo group.	*The Treatment Group:* (38 subjects) received ultrasound (frequency 1 MHz, pulsed 1:4, intensity of 1–2 W/cm^2) applied for 5 to 10 min to the lateral epicondyle. Each participant received 12 treatments. *The Placebo Group:* (38 subjects) received placebo ultrasound for the same period of time.	Patients were assessed for pain, weightlifting and grip strength.	24 patients (63%) treated with ultrasound and 11 (29%) given placebo ultrasound showed a satisfactory outcome on objective testing both at the end of treatment and during further follow-up.

Authors	Aim of study	Numbers	Methods	Assessment	Results
Brosseau et al (2001)	To assess the effectiveness and side-effects of ultrasound therapy for treating patellofemoral knee pain syndrome.		The authors undertook a systematic search of the literature. Only one study, a randomised controlled trial (RCT), met their inclusion criteria and was reviewed by the authors.		The authors conclude that ultrasound therapy was not shown to have a clinically important effect on pain relief for people with patellofemoral pain syndrome.
Busse et al (2002)		Six studies were reviewed by the authors.	The authors conducted a systematic review and meta-analysis of RCTs to determine whether low-intensity pulsed ultrasound therapy affects the time to fracture healing. Six studies met their inclusion criteria and underwent review. Of the six studies, three were excluded from the final analysis. The pooled results from the remaining three studies showed that the time to healing was significantly shorter in the groups receiving low-intensity pulsed ultrasound treatment than in the control groups.		The authors conclude that ultrasound therapy may be beneficial to fracture healing.

Authors	Aim of study	Numbers	Methods	Assessment	Results
Downing & Weinstein (1986)	To determine whether the addition of ultrasound could further decrease pain and increase range of movement in patients receiving the usual courses of exercises and NSAIDs or exercises in patients with supraspinatus tendonitis, subacromial bursitis and adhesive capsulitis (SSA).	20 patients with SSA were randomly assigned to an active ultrasound group or a 'sham' ultrasound group.	The active group (11 subjects) received ultrasound (frequency 1 MHz, continuous, intensity 1.2 W/cm^2) applied for 6 min to the shoulder region, 3 times a week for 4 weeks (12 treatments). The 'sham' group (9 subjects) had the same set-up but the power was turned off. Home exercises were given to each patient.	Pain, range of movement and function were assessed before and after treatment.	No significant difference existed between sham and active ultrasound groups.

Authors	Aim of study	Numbers	Methods	Assessment	Results
Draper et al (1995)	To plot the rate of temperature increase during ultrasound treatments delivered at various intensities and frequencies.	24 students participated in the study and were allocated to two groups.	*Group 1:* (12 subjects) had two thermistors (measuring muscle temperature) inserted into the muscle belly of the triceps surae muscle to a depth of 2.5 cm and 5.0 cm. Each subject then received a total of 4, 10-min ultrasound treatments (frequency 1 MHz, continuous mode), one each at 0.5, 1.0, 1.5 and 2.0 W/cm². The temperature was measured every 30 s. *Group 2:* (12 subjects) had two thermistors (measuring muscle temperature) inserted into the muscle belly of the triceps surae muscle to a depth of 0.8 cm and 1.6 cm. Each subject then received a total of 4, 10-min ultrasound treatments (frequency 3 MHz, continuous mode), one each at 0.5, 1.0, 1.5 and 2.0 W/cm². The temperature was measured every 30 s.	The temperature of the muscle was measured by inserting two, 23-guage thermistor needles. Temperature was recorded every 30 s.	No significant difference was found in the rate of heating at the two depths within the same frequency and dose levels. On average, the rate of temperature increase/min at the two depths of the 1 MHz frequency was: 0.04°C at 0.5 W/cm²; 0.16°C at 1.0 W/cm²; 0.33°C at 1.5 W/cm²; and 0.38°C at 2.0 W/cm². The rate of temperature increase/min at the two depths of the 3 MHz frequency was: 0.3°C at 0.5 W/cm²; 0.58°C at 1.0 W/cm²; 0.89°C at 1.5 W/cm²; and 1.4°C at 2.0 W/cm².

Authors	Aim of study	Numbers	Methods	Assessment	Results
Eriksson et al (1991)	To determine the effects of ultrasound on the healing of chronic leg ulcers.	38 patients with venous leg ulcers were randomly assigned to a treatment group or a control group.	*The Treatment Group*: (12 subjects) received a standard therapeutic regimen and ultrasound (frequency 1 MHz, intensity of 1.0 W/cm^2) for 10 min, applied to the ulcer surface area and surrounding tissue, twice weekly for 8 weeks. *The Control Group*: (13 subjects) received the standard regimen and placebo ultrasound, twice weekly for 8 weeks.	A baseline tracing of the ulcer area was carried out prior to the study and at the end of the study, using a computer graphics programme.	There were no significant differences in the proportion of healed ulcers or ulcer area in the ultrasound group compared with the placebo group. The authors did note that there was a tendency that the ultrasound was more effective than the placebo.
Everett et al (1992)	To determine the effectiveness of ultrasound in the treatment of persistent postnatal perineal pain and dyspareunia.	69 patients with perineal pain were randomly assigned to a treatment group or a control group.	*The Treatment Group*: (37 subjects) received ultrasound (frequency of 3 MHz, pulsed 1:1, intensity of 0.5 W/cm^2, giving an average power of 0.2 W/cm^2 for 5 minutes), 3 times weekly for 8 treatments. (KY jelly was used as a coupling medium.) *The Control Group*: (32 subjects) received 'sham' ultrasound.	The patients were assessed for perineal pain and dyspareunia, 6 weeks after recruitment, using a self-administered questionnaire.	Women in both groups improved over the course of the study.

Authors	Aim of study	Numbers	Methods	Assessment	Results
Gam & Johannsen (1995)	The aim of the paper was to present the result of a meta-analysis on the effectiveness of therapeutic ultrasound in the treatment of pain in musculoskeletal disorders.		The authors reviewed 22 papers and concluded that the use of ultrasound in the treatment of musculoskeletal disorders was based on empirical evidence, lacking firm evidence from well-designed controlled studies.		
Grant et al (1989)	To determine the effectiveness of ultrasound and pulsed electromagnetic energy (PEME) treatment for perineal trauma.	414 patients with perineal trauma were randomly allocated to one of four groups.	*Group 1:* (140 subjects) received active ultrasound (frequency 3 MHz, pulsed 1:4, intensity of 0.5 W/cm^2) for 2 min to each area of trauma. *Group 2:* (135 subjects) received active PEME (pulse frequency 100 Hz, pulse width of 65 μs) for 10 min to the area of trauma. *Groups 3 and 4:* (139 subjects) received 'sham' ultrasound or PEME.	Patients were assessed for pain using the visual analogue scale (VAS), extent of oedema, bruising and haemorrhoids and any analgesia over the course of the treatment. A further assessment was undertaken after 10 days and then by questionnaire 3 months postpartum.	There were no clear differences between the groups in outcome either immediately after treatment, or 10 days or 3 months postpartum.

Authors	Aim of study	Numbers	Methods	Assessment	Results
Gray et al (1995)	To evaluate and compare the effects of four different electrotherapy modalities: shortwave diathermy, megapulse (pulsed shortwave diathermy), ultrasound and laser therapy on patients with temporomandibular pain dysfunction (TMPDS).	139 patients with TMPDS were randomly allocated into one of five groups.	*Group 1:* (27 subjects) received shortwave diathermy at a mild setting for 10 min. *Group 2:* (27 subjects) received megapulse (pulsed shortwave diathermy) (pulse frequency 100 Hz, pulse duration 60 µs) for 20 min. *Group 3:* (30 subjects) received ultrasound (3 MHz, pulsed 2:1, intensity of 0.25 W/cm^2) for 2 min. *Group 4:* (29 subjects) received laser therapy (wavelength 904 nm, dosage of 4 J/cm^2) for 3 min. *Group 5:* (26 subjects) received placebo treatment with one of the above modalities. All participants received treatment 3 times a week for 4 weeks.	Assessment of improvement was made objectively on the basis of a total symptom profile. Those symptoms recorded pre- and post-treatment were muscle tenderness, joint tenderness, joint sounds and joint tenderness on direct palpation. Range of movement (ROM) was measured and the subjective improvement was recorded on the basis of the patients' report on their overall state (worse, unchanged, variable, much better or cured).	At the time of the first review, 7 days after the completion of treatment, there was no significant difference in the success rate between any of the treatment groups or between the treated and placebo groups. At the final review, at 3 months, a definite and significant difference between the treated and placebo groups had emerged.

Authors	Aim of study	Numbers	Methods	Assessment	Results
Holmes & Rudland (1991)		18 studies were reviewed by the authors.	The authors conducted a systematic review of the literature to determine the effectiveness of ultrasound therapy in the treatment of soft tissue injuries. 18 studies were identified and underwent review. These studies fall broadly into three categories: investigation of therapeutic ultrasound in isolation; investigations of ultrasound in combination with other treatments; and those that have compared combination treatments, including and excluding ultrasound.		Only 3 studies emerged without methodological flaws. The authors conclude that the need to design well-controlled and discriminative studies is of paramount importance.
Kitchen & Partridge (1990)	This excellent paper covers the physiological effects and hazards of ultrasound and the efficacy of ultrasound.				

Authors	Aim of study	Numbers	Methods	Assessment	Results
Lundeberg et al (1988)	To compare the effects of continuous ultrasound, placebo ultrasound and untreated controls in patients suffering from epicondylalgia (tennis elbow).	99 patients with epicondylalgia (tennis elbow) were randomly allocated to three groups.	*Group 1:* (33 subjects) received ultrasound (frequency 1 MHz, continuous, intensity of 1.0 W/cm^2) for 10 min, twice weekly for 5 weeks (10 treatments). *Group 2:* (33 subjects) received placebo ultrasound and were instructed to rest. *Group 3:* (33 subjects) received only instruction to rest.	Patients were assessed for pain, using the visual analogue scale (VAS), pain using a test resisting wrist extension compared with the normal wrist, a weight test to assess the ability to lift weights and grip strength.	There was no significant difference in recovery in patients receiving the active ultrasound or placebo ultrasound treatment.
Marks et al (2000)	The authors conducted a systematic review of the literature to determine the effectiveness of ultrasound therapy in decreasing pain and improving the function of people with osteoarthritis (OA) of the knee.	Five studies were reviewed by the authors.	Five studies were identified and reviewed by the authors. All were deemed to have methodological inaccuracies.		

Authors	Aim of study	Numbers	Methods	Assessment	Results
Maxwell (1992)			This paper reviews the ways in which ultrasound may affect inflammation and repair. The author concludes by stating that ultrasound may potentiate or inhibit inflammation due to its capacity to generate free radicals.		Either directly or by way of these chemical species, ultrasound can influence blood flow, the mediation of inflammation, leukocyte migration and function, angiogenesis, collagen synthesis and maturation, and scar formation.
Nyanzi et al (1999)	To investigate the role of ultrasound compared with placebo in the management of recent sprains of the ankle.	51 patients with inversion injuries of the ankle were randomly allocated to an active treatment group or a placebo group.	Group 1: (26 subjects) received ultrasound (frequency 3 MHz, pulsed 1:4, intensity of 0.25 W/cm^2) for 10 min, on 3 consecutive days. Group 2: (25 subjects) received placebo ultrasound.	Patients were assessed for pain, using the visual analogue scale (VAS), ankle swelling (tape measure), ankle movements (goniometer) and weight bearing (scales). Patients were assessed at every visit and 14 days after the last session.	Patients in both the ultrasound and placebo groups improved during the study.

Authors	Aim of study	Numbers	Methods	Assessment	Results
Nykänen (1995)	To determine the effect of pulsed ultrasound on shoulder pain.	72 patients with painful shoulders were randomly assigned to two groups.	*Group 1*: (35 subjects) received pulsed ultrasound (frequency 1 MHz, pulsed 1:4, intensity of 1 W/cm^2) for 10 min and a rehabilitation programme, for 10–12 treatments. *Group 2*: (37 subjects) received placebo ultrasound and a rehabilitation programme, for 10–12 treatments.	The patients were assessed for range of movement (abduction) using a goniometer, and pain. Patients were assessed before treatment and at discharge.	After the treatment period, the same degree of favourable progress was seen in both ultrasound and placebo groups, without significant differences between the groups.
Robertson (2002)	To document the dosage details and treatment responses in RCTs of ultrasound to treat pain and to promote soft tissue healing.	24 studies were reviewed by the authors.	The author conducted a systematic review of RCTs, which used ultrasound to treat people with pain or soft tissue lesions. 24 studies were identified and analysed to ascertain all details of the dosage and outcomes. These were reviewed by the author.		The author concludes that the study was unable to identify a relationship between the dosage and outcomes by analysing the RCTs.

Authors	Aim of study	Numbers	Methods	Assessment	Results
Robertson & Baker (2001)		10 studies were reviewed by the authors.	The authors conducted a systematic review of RCTs to determine the effectiveness of ultrasound therapy for treating people with pain, musculoskeletal injuries, and soft tissue lesions. 35 studies were identified, but only 10 were deemed to have acceptable methodology. These were reviewed by the authors.		The authors conclude by saying there is still little evidence of the clinical effectiveness of therapeutic ultrasound as currently used by therapists to treat people with pain and musculoskeletal injuries and to promote soft tissue healing.
Roebroeck et al (1998)	The results showed that Dutch therapists applied ultrasound for recent soft tissue injuries, mainly aiming to reduce pain and swelling. Ultrasound was combined quite frequently with massage.				
Speed (2001)	This paper reviews the scientific basis for the use of therapeutic ultrasound in soft tissue lesions and the existing evidence relating to its clinical effect. The paper states that therapeutic ultrasound is one of the most common treatments used in the management of soft tissue lesions. The author discusses the characteristics of therapeutic ultrasound, the physiological effects of ultrasound and the clinical evidence.				

Authors	Aim of study	Numbers	Methods	Assessment	Results
Ter Haar (1999)	This paper is a review of therapeutic ultrasound. The author states that the intention of the lower intensity treatments is to stimulate normal physiological processes to injury, or to accelerate some processes such as the transport of drugs across the skin. She discusses the physiological basis for therapeutic ultrasound: the thermal and non-thermal effects. The use of ultrasound in the treatment of soft tissue injuries and bone healing is explained.				
van der Windt et al (1999)	The objective of the review was to evaluate the effectiveness of ultrasound therapy in the treatment of musculoskeletal disorders.	38 studies were reviewed by the authors.	The author conducted a systematic review of RCTs. 38 studies were reviewed, evaluating the effects of ultrasound for lateral epicondylitis, shoulder pain, degenerative rheumatic disorders, ankle distortions, temporomandibular pain and a variety of other disorders.		The authors conclude by stating that there seems to be little evidence to support the use of ultrasound therapy in the treatment of musculoskeletal disorders.

Authors	Aim of study	Numbers	Methods	Assessment	Results
Vasseljen (1992)	To compare the effect of low-level laser therapy to a treatment of pulsed ultrasound and deep frictions for tennis elbow.	30 patients with tennis elbow were randomly assigned to two groups.	*Group 1*: (15 subjects) received gallium-arsenide (GaAs) laser (wavelength 904 nm, giving a dose on the skin surface of 3.5 J/cm^2) 3 times weekly for 8 treatments. *Group 2*: (15 subjects) received pulsed ultrasound (frequency 1 MHz, intensity of 1.5 W/cm^2) for 7 min plus deep frictions for 10 min to extensor carpi radialis brevis.	Measurements assessed were grip strength, weight test, wrist flexion, visual analogue scale (VAS) and patient assessment.	Laser therapy and pulsed ultrasound and deep frictions had a significant effect on the symptoms of tennis elbow. Laser was no better than pulsed ultrasound and deep frictions.
Warden et al (1999)	This paper focuses on the safe application and effects of appropriately dosaged ultrasound when applied during fracture repair. When applied to fresh fractures, ultrasound (using a specialised ultrasonic unit) has been shown to substantially accelerate the rate of repair. These machines use an intensity below 0.1 W/cm^2, which cannot be produced by a conventional ultrasound unit.				
Watson (2000)	The author discusses current concepts in electrotherapy, the electrical potential of the cell, high and low energy approaches, frequency and amplitude windows and modalities. The sections on 'interferential' and 'ultrasound' are particularly informative.				

Authors	Aim of study	Numbers	Methods	Assessment	Results
Zammit & Herrington (2005)	To determine the efficacy of ultrasound therapy in the management of acute lateral sprains of the ankle joint.	29 patients with acute lateral ligament sprains of the ankle were randomly assigned to three treatment groups.	*Group 1:* (10 subjects) received an ice pack and ultrasound (3 MHz, pulsed 1:4, intensity of 0.25 W/cm² for 10 min for three treatments and pulsed 1:2, intensity of 0.5 W/cm² for 6 min for a further three treatments). *Group 2:* (10 subjects) received an ice pack and ultrasound, which was applied identically to the above, but without the emitter switched on. *Group 3:* (9 subjects) received an ice pack. All participants were supplied with a Tubigrip, given specific exercises and advised to use ice at home.	Patients were assessed for pain (using the visual analogue scale), swelling (tape measure), range of ankle movements (goniometer) and postural stability (balance error scoring system).	No statistical differences were detected between treatment groups in pain, swelling, range of movement and postural stability.

REFERENCES

Baker K G, Robertson V J, Duck F A 2001 A review of therapeutic ultrasound: Biophysical effects. Physical Therapy 81:1351–1358

Binder A, Hodge G, Greenwood A et al 1985 Is therapeutic ultrasound effective in treating soft tissue lesions? British Medical Journal 290:512–514

Brosseau L, Casimiro L, Judd M G et al 2001 Therapeutic ultrasound for treating patellofemoral pain syndrome (Review). Issue 4. The Cochrane Database of Systematic Reviews

Busse J W, Bhandari M, Kulkarni A V et al 2002 The effect of low-intensity pulsed ultrasound on time to fracture healing: a meta-analysis. Canadian Medical Association Journal 166:437–441

Downing D S, Weinstein A 1986 Ultrasound therapy of subacromial bursitis: A double blind trial. Physical Therapy 66:194–199

Draper D O, Castel J C, Castel D 1995 Rate of temperature increase in human muscle during 1 MHz and 3 MHz continuous ultrasound. Journal of Orthopaedic and Sports Physical Therapy 22:142–150

Eriksson S V, Lundeberg T, Malm M 1991 A placebo controlled trial of ultrasound therapy in chronic leg ulceration. Scandinavian Journal of Rehabilitation Medicine 23:211–213

Everett T, McIntosh J, Grant A 1992 Ultrasound therapy for persistent post-natal perineal pain and dyspareunia: A randomised placebo-controlled trial. Physiotherapy 78:263–267

Gam A N, Johannsen F 1995 Ultrasound therapy in musculoskeletal disorders: a meta-analysis. Pain 63:85–91

Grant A, Sleep J, McIntosh J, Ashurst H 1989 Ultrasound and pulsed electromagnetic energy treatment for perineal trauma. A randomized placebo-controlled trial. British Journal of Obstetrics and Gynaecology 9:434–439

Gray R J, Quayle A A, Hall C A, Schofield M A 1995 Temporomandibular pain dysfunction: can electrotherapy help? Physiotherapy 81:47–51

Holmes M A M, Rudland J R 1991 Clinical trials of ultrasound treatment in soft tissue injury: A review and critique. Physiotherapy Theory and Practice 7:163–175

Kitchen S, Partridge C 1990 A review of therapeutic ultrasound. Physiotherapy 76:593–600

Lundeberg T, Abrahamsson P, Haker E 1988 A comparative study of continuous ultrasound, placebo ultrasound and rest in epicondylalgia. Scandinavian Journal of Rehabilitation Medicine 20:99–101

Marks R, Ghanagaraja S, Ghassemi M 2000 Ultrasound for osteoarthritis of the knee: A systematic review. Physiotherapy 86:452–463

Maxwell L 1992 Therapeutic ultrasound: Its effects on the cellular and molecular mechanisms of inflammation and repair. Physiotherapy 78:421–426

Nyanzi C S, Langridge J, Heyworth J R C et al 1999 Randomized controlled study of ultrasound therapy in the management of acute lateral ligament sprains of the ankle joint. Clinical Rehabilitation 13:16–22

Nykänen M 1995 Pulsed ultrasound treatment of the painful shoulder: a randomized, double-blind, placebo-controlled study. Scandinavian Journal of Rehabilitation Medicine 27:105–108

Robertson V J 2002 Dosage and treatment response in randomized clinical trials of therapeutic ultrasound. Physical Therapy in Sport 3:124–133

Robertson V J, Baker K J 2001 A review of therapeutic ultrasound: effectiveness studies. Physical Therapy 81:1339–1350

Robertson V, Ward A, Low J et al 2006 Electrotherapy explained: principles and practice, 4th edn. Elsevier Science, Oxford

Roebroeck M E, Dekker J, Oostendorp R A B 1998 The use of therapeutic ultrasound by physical therapists in Dutch primary health care. Physical Therapy 78:470–478

Speed C A 2001 Therapeutic ultrasound in soft tissue lesions. Rheumatology 40:1331–1336

Ter Haar G 1999 Therapeutic ultrasound. European Journal of Ultrasound 9:3–9

van der Windt D A W M, van der Heijden G J M G, van den-Berg S G M et al 1999 Ultrasound therapy for musculoskeletal disorders: a systematic review. Pain 81:257–271

Vasseljen O 1992 Low-level laser versus traditional physiotherapy in the treatment of tennis elbow. Physiotherapy 78:329–334

Warden S J, Bennell K L, McMeeken J M et al 1999 Can conventional therapeutic ultrasound units be used to accelerate fracture repair? Physical Therapy Review 4:117–126

Watson T 2000 The role of electrotherapy in contemporary physiotherapy practice. Manual Therapy 5:132–141

Young S 2002 Ultrasound therapy. In: Kitchen S (ed) Electrotherapy: evidence-based practice. Churchill Livingstone, London, p 211–230

Zammit E, Herrington L 2005 Ultrasound therapy in the management of acute lateral ligament sprains of the ankle joint. Physical Therapy in Sport 6:116–121

CHAPTER 10

Laser therapy

PRODUCTION

LASER is an acronym for **L**ight **A**mplification by **S**timulated **E**mission of **R**adiation. The laser medium will either be gaseous (helium-neon, HeNe), semiconductor based gallium-arsenide (GaAs), or gallium-aluminium-arsenide (GaAlAs). The helium-neon laser has a wavelength of 632.8 nm and the gallium-arsenide laser has a wavelength of 904 nm.

In a laser, when electrons are stimulated at a rapid rate, resultant photons are aligned in a reflecting chamber or resonant cavity, composed of mirrors. Photons hit a semi-permeable silver resonating mirror and are reflected back to a reflecting mirror. This back-and-forth reflection of photons intensifies the light until the chamber cannot contain the energy level. The photons are then ejected through the semi-permeable mirror and out through the diode in the applicator head.

Light is part of the electromagnetic spectrum and light generated by laser sources is situated in the visible part of the spectrum (400–700 nm), in particular to the red (630–700 nm) and also to the near infrared part of the spectrum from 750–950 nm.

CHARACTERISTICS OF LASER RADIATION

MONOCHROMATICITY

The light produced by a laser is of a single colour; the radiation emitted being of a single wavelength. The wavelength determines the specific therapeutic effects produced by the laser due to the specific biomolecules absorbing the radiation.

COLLIMATION

The rays of light or photons produced by the laser are practically parallel, with almost no divergence occurring.

COHERENCE

The light emitted is in phase, which means that the troughs and peaks of the emitted waves match perfectly in time (temporal coherence) and space (spatial coherence).

DOSAGE AND IRRADIATION PARAMETERS

POWER OUTPUT

The power output is usually expressed in milliwatts (mW) and is usually fixed. Pulsing can have an effect on the power output of the unit. The trend is for higher output devices (30–200 mW) because they can deliver a specified treatment in a shorter period of time.

POWER DENSITY (IRRADIANCE)

This is the power per unit area (mW/cm^2).

ENERGY

This is expressed in joules (J) and is usually specified per point irradiated. It is calculated by multiplying the power output in watts by the time of irradiation in seconds. Thus a 30 mW (0.03 W) device applied for 1 min (60 s) will deliver 1.8 J of energy.

ENERGY DENSITY

This is expressed in joules per unit area (J/cm^2). Energy density is usually calculated by dividing the energy delivered (in joules) by the spot size of the treatment unit (in cm).

PULSE REPETITION RATE

For pulsed units, the pulse repetition rate is expressed in hertz (Hz, pulses per second).

APPLICATION

Due to the potential harmful effects to the retina and the ability of the laser beam to reflect from most surfaces it is generally accepted to use the laser in a separate room, where possible. Warning signs must be placed on the door or on the curtains of the treatment area. Both patient and operator and anyone else present in the treatment room must wear dark protective glasses, specific to the wavelength of the laser being used.

Laser therapy

The laser machine is set up as follows:

1. Position the patient in a comfortable position with the area exposed.
2. Re-check for any contraindications to treatment and gain informed consent.
3. Screw the probe into the unit.
4. Insert the security key and turn clockwise. The green light should illuminate.
5. Place the probe in the IR sensor and depress the probe switch. If all is well, the red light will come on.
6. Select the appropriate pulse rate frequency (PRF) setting.
7. Select the treatment time.
8. Place the probe at right angles to the area to be treated and press into the tissue.
9. Depress the probe switch to start treatment, a yellow light should appear and a low level audible signal will be heard.
10. At the end of treatment, an audible signal will be heard.
11. Release the probe switch and turn the key off and remove it from the machine.
12. Check the patient's skin for any adverse effects to treatment.

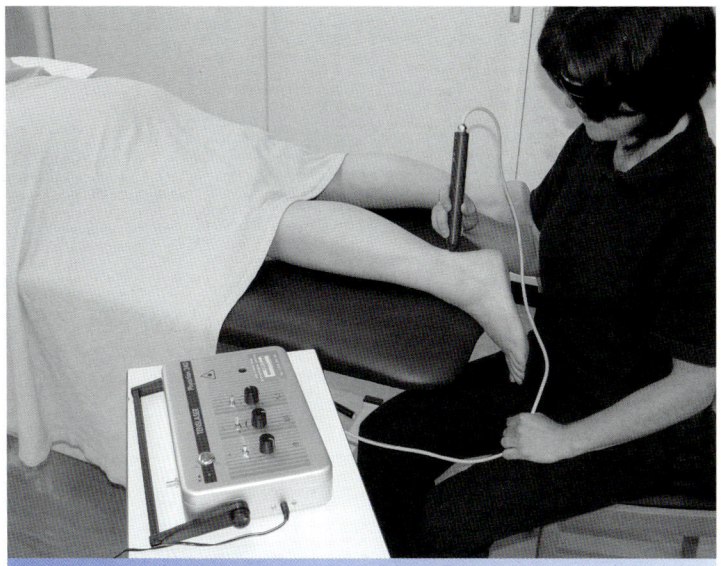

Figure 10.1 Application of laser to the Achilles tendon. The probe is at right angles (90°) to the area to be treated.

ADAPTATIONS

Low level laser therapy can also be administered with a cluster head attachment to enable treatment of a larger area.

Biostimulating effects
Alteration in membrane potentials and enzyme activity
Phagocytosis, neurotransmitter release, and collagen, protein and ribonucleic acid (RNA) synthesis and an improved circulation
May enhance pain relief, resolution of inflammation and swelling, collagen synthesis and enhance chondrocyte activity
Pain relief may occur due to stimulation of peripheral nerves, increase in serotonin metabolism
May also be due to neural repair, a reduction in prostaglandin synthesis, and an improved circulation
May have a stimulating effect on fibroblast proliferation and wound healing.

Clinical application
Stimulation of wound healing
Treatment of various arthritic conditions
Treatment of soft tissue injuries
Relief of pain.

Dangers
Damage to the retina of the eye.

Contraindications
Direct treatment to the eye
Areas of haemorrhage
Radiotherapy
Active cancer
Treatment over a pregnant uterus.

Treatment only with caution
Areas of hypoaesthesia
Infected tissue (infective dermatitis)
Treatment over epiphyseal lines in children
Treatment over the sympathetic ganglion, the vagus nerve and the cardiac region of the thorax in patients with heart disease
Patients with obtunded reflexes

Patients with cognitive difficulties
Over photosensitive areas/sensitised skin
Reproductive organs.

(See Robertson et al 2006 and Baxter 2002.)

Notes

Laser therapy 219

Treatment record

Table 10.1 *OBSERVATIONAL/REFLECTIVE CHECKLIST*

	Observation	Y/N	Comments
Introduction	Did the therapist introduce him/herself?	☐	☐
	Was an explanation of the procedure given?	☐	☐
	Was the explanation clear and succinct?	☐	☐
	Were the possible dangers highlighted?	☐	☐
	Was consent obtained?	☐	☐
Comfort and safety	Was the patient comfortable?	☐	☐
	Was the therapist's posture compromised?	☐	☐
	Was the position safe for both parties?	☐	☐
	Was the modality applied with due care and attention?	☐	☐
Technique	Were the contraindications checked?	☐	☐
	Were the appropriate tests performed prior to treatment?	☐	☐
	Was an explanation of the physiological effects of the technique offered to the patient?	☐	☐
	Was this explanation accurate?	☐	☐
	Was the technique/modality applied correctly?	☐	☐
	Were the correct times and settings used?	☐	☐
	Was the skin checked after the treatment for adverse effects?	☐	☐

Table 10.2 SUMMARY OF STUDIES INVESTIGATING THE EFFECTIVENESS OF LASER THERAPY

Authors	Aim of study	Numbers	Methods	Assessment	Results
Ashford et al (1999)	This paper describes two case studies, showing that it is the length of time that laser therapy is used that can have a significant impact on ulcer size.	Two patients with chronic venous leg ulcers.	Both patients had participated in a randomised crossover trial and at the end of the trial (14 weeks), their ulcers had shown no improvement in size reduction. Both patients received a further course of gallium-aluminium-arsenide (GaAlAs) laser (cluster probe containing 41 diodes, wavelength 660–950 nm, pulsing frequency 5 KHz, average density 4.2 J/cm^2) irradiated for 120 s, twice weekly for 20 weeks.	The size of the ulcer was traced 3 times onto an acetate sheet and photographed every 2 weeks.	After 20 weeks of active treatment, one patient had gained a 78% reduction in ulcer size and the other patient had gained a 91% reduction in ulcer size.
Baxter et al (1991)	To assess the current clinical practice of low level laser therapy (LLLT) in Northern Ireland.	116 physiotherapists participated in the study.	Questionnaires were sent to physiotherapy departments in Northern Ireland.		LLLT has become a popular treatment modality. It is used to treat conditions such as: soft tissue injuries (muscle tears, haematomas and

Authors	Aim of study	Numbers	Methods	Assessment	Results
					tendonitis, rheumatoid arthritis, shingles, postoperative wounds and various types of ulcers and burns. 94% of respondents were concerned with the lack of information on treatment parameters.
Chow & Barnsley (2005)	To determine the efficacy of low level laser therapy (LLLT) in the treatment of neck pain through a systematic review of the literature.	Five studies were reviewed by the authors.	The authors undertook a systematic review of the literature. Five RCT studies were reviewed by the authors.	Significant positive effects were reported in four of the five trials in which infrared wavelengths of 780 nm, 810–830 nm, 904 nm and 1064 nm were used.	The authors conclude that LLLT appears to be efficacious for the treatment of neck pain with limited evidence being provided from the reviewed trials.

Authors	Aim of study	Numbers	Methods	Assessment	Results
de Abreu Venancio et al (2005)	To evaluate the effect of low intensity laser therapy (LILT) on relieving pain and improving function in arthrogenic temporo-mandibular disorder (TMD) patients.	30 patients with TMD were randomly assigned to two groups.	*Group 1:* (15 subjects) received gallium-aluminium-arsenide (GaAlAs) laser (wavelength 780 nm, 30 mW, energy density of 6.3 J/cm^2) for 10 s, twice a week for 3 weeks, at 3 points on each temporomandibular joint. *Group 2:* (15 subjects) received inactive laser (placebo) to the same 3 points.	Patients were assessed for pain, using the visual analogue scale (VAS), pain pressure threshold (PPT), using an algometer and measurement of mandibular dysfunction. Each patient was evaluated immediately before the 1st, 3rd and 5th treatment sessions and after 15, 30 and 60 days post-treatment.	There was a significant reduction in pain for both the experimental group and the control group ($p < 0.001$). There was not a significant difference in PPT or measurement of mandibular dysfunction.
de Bie et al (1998a)	To test the efficacy of low-level laser therapy on lateral ankle sprains as an addition to a standard treatment regimen.	217 patients with acute lateral ankle sprains, were randomly assigned to three groups.	*Group 1:* (74 subjects) received gallium-arsenide (GaAs) laser (wavelength 904 nm, with 25 W peak power, pulse duration of 200 nsec, an irradiation area of 1 cm^2, and an energy density of 0.07 J/cm^2). *Group 2:* (72 subjects) received the same laser treatment but at a frequency of 5000 Hz, giving an energy density of 0.7 J/cm^2.	Patients were assessed for pain, VAS, function and limitation in activities of daily living.	Neither high- nor low-dose laser therapy was effective in the treatment of lateral ankle sprains.

Authors	Aim of study	Numbers	Methods	Assessment	Results
			Group 3: (71 subjects) received placebo laser, energy density 0.0 J/cm^2. Every patient received 200 s of laser therapy, involving 12 treatments over a 4-week period.		
de Bie et al (1998b)	This systematic review was undertaken to assess the effectiveness of 904 nm low level laser therapy in musculoskeletal disorders.		This paper is a review of laboratory and clinical research studies that have investigated the effects of therapeutic modalities on wound healing. A critical appraisal of the clinical research available that supports the use of each of the modalities to treat chronic wounds is also provided.		
Franek et al (2002)	To determine whether low output laser enhances the healing of crural ulcers.	65 patients with crural ulcerations were randomly allocated into three groups.	Group 1: (21 subjects) received compressive therapy, pharmacological treatment and gallium-aluminium-arsenide (GaAlAs) laser (wavelength 810 nm, continuous, 65 mW, average dose of 4 J/cm^2). The laser was wired to a scanner.		There was no significant impact of laser therapy on the healing of the ulcers.

Authors	Aim of study	Numbers	Methods	Assessment	Results
Gray et al (1995)	To evaluate and compare the effects of four different electrotherapy modalities, namely shortwave diathermy, megapulse (pulsed shortwave diathermy), ultrasound and laser therapy on patients with temporomandibular pain dysfunction (TMPDS).	139 patients with TMPDS were randomly allocated into five groups.	*Group 1:* (27 subjects) received shortwave diathermy at a mild setting for 10 min. *Group 2:* (27 subjects) received megapulse (pulsed shortwave diathermy) (pulse frequency 100 Hz, pulse duration 60 μs) for 20 min. *Group 3:* (30 subjects) received ultrasound (3 MHz, pulsed 2:1, intensity of 0.25 W/cm^2) for 2 min. *Group 4:* (29 subjects) received laser therapy (wavelength 904 nm, dosage of 4 J/cm^2) for 3 min. *Group 5:* (26 subjects) received placebo treatment with one of the above modalities. All participants received treatment 3 times a week for 4 weeks.	Assessment of improvement was made objectively on the basis of a total symptom profile. Those symptoms recorded pre-and post-treatment were muscle tenderness, joint sounds and joint tenderness on direct palpation. Range of movement (ROM) was measured and the subjective improvement was recorded on the basis of the patients' report on their overall state (worse, unchanged, variable, much better or cured).	At the time of the first review, 7 days after the completion of treatment, there was no significant difference in the success rate between any of the treatment groups or between the treated and placebo groups. At the final review, at 3 months, a definite and significant difference between the treated and placebo groups had emerged.

Group 2: (22 subjects) received compressive therapy, pharmacological treatment and placebo laser.

Group 3: (22 subjects) received compressive therapy and pharmacological treatment.

Authors	Aim of study	Numbers	Methods	Assessment	Results
Gupta et al (1998)	To determine the effects of low energy photon therapy (LEPT) on venous leg ulcers.	Nine patients with 12 ulcers were randomly allocated into two groups.	*The Treatment Group*: received infrared laser (wavelength 880 nm, 12 mW, energy density 4 J/cm^2, pulse frequency 4 Hz and covering an area of 4 cm^2), for 30 s to the periphery of the wound. A second probe (wavelength 660 nm, 6 mW, continuous, energy density 4 J/cm^2, and covering an area of 6 × 10 cm^2), for 180 s to the bed of the ulcer. *The Placebo Group*: received sham therapy from the same devices. All the participants were treated 3 times a week for 10 weeks (30 treatments).		The percentage of the initial area remaining unhealed in the LEPT and placebo groups was 24% and 85%, respectively ($p = 0.0008$).
Houghton (1999)	To review the effects of therapeutic modalities on wound healing.		This paper is a review of laboratory and clinical research studies that have investigated the effects of therapeutic modalities on wound healing. A critical appraisal of the clinical research available that supports the use of each of the modalities to treat chronic wounds has also been provided.		

Laser therapy

Authors	Aim of study	Numbers	Methods	Assessment	Results
Irvine et al (2004)	To determine the effects of low-level laser therapy (LLLT) on carpal tunnel syndrome.	15 patients with mild to moderate carpal tunnel syndrome were randomly assigned to two groups.	*Group 1:* (7 subjects) received gallium-aluminium-arsenide (GaAlAs) laser (wavelength 860 nm, emitted a 60 mW beam at an intensity of 3 J/cm^2, delivering a total of 6 J/cm^2 in 15 s) 3 times a week for 5 weeks to 20 sites over and surrounding the carpal tunnel. *Group 2:* (8 subjects) received a similar regime with a 'sham' laser.	Each participant was assessed using the Levine Carpal Tunnel Syndrome Questionnaire, electrophysiological data and the Purdue pegboard test.	There was a significant symptomatic improvement in both the control ($p = 0.034$) and treatment ($p = 0.043$) groups. LLT was no more effective in the reduction of symptoms than the sham treatment.
Kitchen & Partridge (1991)	A review of low level laser therapy		This is an excellent, extensive review paper.		

Authors	Aim of study	Numbers	Methods	Assessment	Results
Kleinman et al (1996)		42 patients with resistant venous ulcers were assigned to two groups.	*Group 1:* (29 subjects) received gallium-arsenide (GaAs) laser (9 diode, continuous, wavelength 785 nm, 6 mW (each diode) for 20 min in a manual scanning mode) applied every other day. *Group 2:* (13 subjects) with multiple wounds received combined helium-neon (HeNe) (wavelength 632.8 nm, 6 mW) laser and gallium-aluminium-arsenide (GaAlAs) infrared laser (wavelength 765 nm, 80 mW) with a pulse rate of 0.1–10 kHz. Each area was irradiated at 4 kHz for 15 min every other day.		Complete wound closure was achieved in 36 of the 42 cases.
Laakso et al (1993)	The purpose of the paper was to clarify some of the parameters of laser which may affect the treatment of patients. The paper discussed the significance of wavelength, power output, dose, pulse frequency, frequency of treatment and potential side-effects.				

Laser therapy

Authors	Aim of study	Numbers	Methods	Assessment	Results
Lagan et al (2002)		15 patients with chronic venous ulcers were assigned to two groups.	Group 1: (8 subjects) received gallium-aluminium-arsenide (GaAlAs) laser (multiwavelength 660–950 mn, 31 diodes, average output 532 mW, pulse frequency 5 kHz, average dosage 12 J/cm^2) once a week for 4 weeks plus a standardised nursing regime. Group 2: (7 subjects) received a 'sham' laser plus the standardised nursing regime.		There was no statistical difference between treatment and placebo groups, but an apparent difference in wound healing rate was noted for the treatment group.
Lundeberg & Malm (1991)	To determine the effect of low-power helium-neon (HeNe) laser treatment on venous leg ulcers.	46 patients with venous leg ulcers were randomly assigned to two groups.	Group 1: received a standard treatment plus HeNe laser (wavelength 632.8, beam power 6 mW, continuous emission, energy density 4 J/cm^2) applied twice a week for 12 weeks. Group 2: received a standard treatment plus placebo laser.		There were no significant differences in the proportion of healed ulcers or ulcer area in the HeNe group compared with the placebo group.

Authors	Aim of study	Numbers	Methods	Assessment	Results
Malm & Lundeberg (1991)	To determine the effect of low power gallium-arsenide (GaAs) laser on healing of venous ulcers.	42 patients with venous leg ulcers were randomly allocated into two groups.	*Group 1:* (21 subjects) received a standard treatment plus GaAs laser (wavelength 904 nm, average output 4 mW, peak power 10 W, pulse frequency 3800 Hz, energy density 1.96 J/cm^2) for 10 min. *Group 2:* (21 subjects) received a standard treatment plus placebo laser.		There were no differences in the results of the two groups.
Marks & de Palma (1999)	To review the clinical efficacy of low power laser therapy in osteoarthritis (OA).	Six studies were reviewed by the author.	This is a very comprehensive paper, discussing the biostimulatory effects of low-level laser therapy, summarising and critically analysing the six studies describing the effects of laser therapy for the treatment of OA.		

Laser therapy

Authors	Aim of study	Numbers	Methods	Assessment	Results
Nussbaum et al (2003)	A review of laser technology and light-tissue interactions as a background to therapeutic application of low intensity lasers and other light sources.		This paper reviews aspects of laser physics, radiometry and photochemistry relevant to the use of low intensity light therapy delivered by lasers. Current theories regarding the biophysical mechanisms of low intensity laser therapy are reviewed. Characteristics of laser radiation such as monochromaticity, coherence, collimation, speckle, beam profile, penetration depth and temporal modulation of irradiation, and the relevance of these factors to photon propagation are explained.		
Pope et al (1995)	To assess the current clinical use of electro-therapeutic modalities in the NHS in England.		Laser units were widely owned and frequently used. 196 respondents owned laser units and only 14 respondents did not use this modality. Out of 88 respondents, almost half (41) used laser 2/3 times a day and a further four respondents used laser daily.		

Authors	Aim of study	Numbers	Methods	Assessment	Results
Saunders (1995)	To determine the efficacy of low-level laser therapy in the treatment of supraspinatus tendinitis.	24 patients with supraspinatus tendinitis were randomly assigned to two groups.	*The Treatment Group:* received infrared laser (wavelength 820 nm, energy density 40 mW, operating at 5000 Hz, producing a dosage of 30 J/cm^2, and giving a 90 s irradiation) to 2 points on the shoulder. Nine treatments were given over a period of 3 weeks. *The Placebo Group:* received a dummy laser.		Laser and advice alleviated the symptoms (pain, tenderness and muscle strength) of supraspinatus tendonitis.
Schindl et al (1999)	To investigate whether low-intensity irradiations were of beneficial effect on long-term ulcers.	20 patients with long-term ulcers participated in the study.	All the participants had previously received 'conventional' treatment without achieving healing. They were all treated with HeNe laser (wavelength 632.8 nm, energy density of 30 J/cm^2) along the wound edge, 3 times weekly, until complete closure of the ulcer occurred.		Complete closure occurred in all cases, within a median of 12.5 weeks (range 4–45 weeks). The authors concluded that healing time correlated with the ulcer cause and size.

Authors	Aim of study	Numbers	Methods	Assessment	Results
Sharma et al (2002)	To evaluate the effect of low level laser therapy using ultrasonography for assessment in de Quervain's tenosynovitis (inflammation of the pollicis tendon sheath).	28 female patients with de Quervain's tenosynovitis were assigned to a treatment or a control group.	*The Treatment Group:* (13 subjects with 15 tendons) received gallium-aluminium-arsenide (GaAlAs) laser (wavelength 830 nm, power 30–40 mw, beam diameter 4 mm, continuous, applied at dosage of 2–4 J/cm² to the treatment area for a maximum of 10 treatments. *The Control Group:* (15 subjects) received 'sham' laser treatment.	Measurements assessed were pain using VAS, pain/tenderness on pressure over the radial styloid, grip strength and pinch test, using a sphygmomanometer, Finkelstein's test and ultrasound scans of the tendon sheaths.	The treatment (laser therapy) group demonstrated a significant increase in grip strength ($p < 0.01$) and pinch grip strength ($p = 0.024$) and a significant decrease in the diameters of the tendon sheaths. The control group demonstrated no improvement.
Sugrue et al (1990)		12 patients with chronic venous ulcers.	All participants had been unresponsive to conservative treatment. Four patients were treated with gallium-aluminium-arsenide (GaAlAs) laser (wavelength 780 nm, continuous output at 0.2 mW, energy was delivered for 15 s/cm²), 3 times weekly for a maximum of 12 weeks. Eight patients were treated with a gallium-arsenide (GaAs) laser (4 probe cluster, wavelength 904 nm, pulsed 4000 Hz, average output 3 mW) for 4 min, to the ulcer, 3 times weekly for a maximum of 12 weeks.		2 ulcers healed completely and there was a 27% reduction in the size of all ulcers.

PRACTICAL ELECTROTHERAPY

Authors	Aim of study	Numbers	Methods	Assessment	Results
Vasseljen (1992)	To compare the effect of low-level laser therapy to a treatment of pulsed ultrasound and deep frictions for tennis elbow.	30 patients with tennis elbow were randomly assigned to two groups.	Group 1: (15 subjects) received gallium-arsenide (GaAs) laser (wavelength 904 nm, giving a dose on the skin surface of 3.5 J/cm^2) 3 times weekly for 8 treatments. Group 2: (15 subjects) received pulsed ultrasound (frequency 1 MHz, intensity of 1.5 W/cm^2 for 7 min) plus deep frictions for 10 min to extensor carpi radialis brevis.	Measurements assessed were grip strength, weight test, wrist flexion, visual analogue scale (VAS) and patient assessment.	Laser therapy and pulsed ultrasound and deep frictions had a significant effect on the symptoms of tennis elbow. Laser was no better than pulsed ultrasound and deep frictions.

REFERENCES

Ashford R, Brown N, Lagan K et al 1999 Low intensity laser therapy for chronic venous ulcers. Nursing Standard 14:66–72

Baxter G D 2002 Low-intensity laser therapy. In: Kitchen S (ed) Electrotherapy: evidence-based practice, 11th edn. Churchill Livingstone, London, p 171–189

Baxter G D, Bell A J, Allen J M et al 1991 Low level laser therapy: current clinical practice in Northern Ireland. Physiotherapy 77:171–178

Chow R T, Barnsley L 2005 Systematic review of the literature of low-level laser therapy (LLLT) in the management of neck pain. Laser in Surgery and Medicine 37:46–52

de Abreu Venancio R, Camparis C M, de Fátima Zanirato R 2005 Low intensity laser therapy in the treatment of temporomandibular disorders: a double-blind study. Journal of Oral Rehabilitation 32:800–807

de Bie R A, de Vet H C, Lenssen T F et al 1998a Low-level laser therapy in ankle sprains: a randomized clinical trial. Archives of Physical Medicine and Rehabilitation 79:1415–1420

de Bie R A, Verhagen A P, Lenssen A F et al 1998b Efficacy of 904 nm laser therapy in the management of musculoskeletal disorders: a systemic review. Physical Therapy Review 3:59–72

Franek A, Król P, Kucharzewski M 2002 Does low output laser stimulation enhance the healing of crural ulceration? Some critical remarks. Medical Engineering Physics 24:607–615

Gray R J M, Hall C A, Quayle A A, Schofield M A 1995 Temporomandibular pain dysfunction: can electrotherapy help? Physiotherapy 81:47–51

Gupta A K, Filonenko N, Salansky N et al 1998 The use of low energy photon therapy (LEPT) in venous leg ulcers: a double-blind, placebo-controlled study. Dermatologic Surgery 24:1383–1386

Houghton P E 1999 Effects of therapeutic modalities on wound healing: a conservative approach to the management of chronic wounds. Physical Therapy Review 4:176–182

Irvine J, Chong S L, Amirjani N et al 2004 Double-blind randomized controlled trial of low-level laser therapy in carpal tunnel syndrome. Muscle and Nerve 30:182–187

Kitchen S S, Partridge C J 1991 A review of low level laser therapy. Physiotherapy 77:161–168

Kleinman Y, Simmer S, Braksma Y et al 1996 Low level laser therapy in patients with venous ulcers: early and long-term outcome. Laser therapy 8:205–208

Laakso L, Richardson C, Cramond T 1993 Factors affecting low level laser therapy. Australian Physiotherapy 39:95–99

Lagan K M, McKenna T, Witherow A et al 2002 Low-intensity laser therapy/combined phototherapy in the management of chronic venous ulceration: a placebo-controlled study. Journal of Clinical Laser Medicine Surgery 20:109–116

Lundeberg T, Malm M 1991 Low-power HeNe laser treatment of venous leg ulcers. Annals of Plastic Surgery 27:537–539

Malm M, Lundeberg T 1991 Effect of low power gallium arsenide laser on healing of venous ulcers. Scandinavian Journal of Plastic and Reconstructive Hand Surgery 25:249–251

Marks R, de Palma F 1999 Clinical efficacy of low power laser therapy in osteoarthritis. Physiotherapy Research International 4:141–157

Nussbaum E L, Baxter G D, Lilge L 2003 A review of laser technology and light-tissue interactions as a background to therapeutic applications of low intensity lasers and other light sources. Physical Therapy Review 8:32–44

Pope G D, Mockett S P, Wright J P 1995 A survey of electrotherapeutic modalities: ownership and use in the NHS in England. Physiotherapy 81:82–91

Robertson V, Ward A, Low J et al 2006 Electrotherapy explained: principles and practice, 4th edn. Elsevier Science, Oxford

Saunders L 1995 The efficacy of low-level laser therapy in supraspinatus tendinitis. Clinical Rehabilitation 9:126–134

Schindl M, Kerschan K, Schindl A et al 1999 Induction of complete wound healing in recalcitrant ulcers by low-intensity laser irradiation depends on ulcer cause and size. Photodermatology, Photoimmunology and Photomedicine 15:18–21

Sharma R, Thukral A, Kumar S et al 2002 Effect of low level lasers in de Quervains tenosynovitis. Physiotherapy 88:730–734

Sugrue M E, Carolan J, Leen E J et al 1990 The use of infrared therapy in the treatment of varicose ulcers. Annals of Vascular Surgery 4:179–181

Vasseljen O 1992 Low-level laser versus traditional physiotherapy in the treatment of tennis elbow. Physiotherapy 78:329–334

APPENDIX 1

Electrical safety

ELECTRIC SHOCK

An electric shock occurs when a current passes through the body. This is a painful stimulation of sensory nerves caused by a sudden flow, cessation or variation in the current passing through the body.

SEVERITY OF SHOCK

The greater the current which passes through the body, the more severe the shock. In accordance with Ohm's law, the magnitude of the current depends upon the electromotive force (EMF) and the resistance. A high EMF is likely to produce a large current. Physiotherapy apparatus is plugged into the mains supply of 240 V at a frequency of 50 Hz. It therefore represents a hazard as a source of electric shock. A high resistance reduces the intensity of the current, so if exposed parts of the circuit are touched with damp hands the shock is more likely to be severe than if the hands are dry.

The severity of the shock also depends on the pathway taken by the current. Strong currents through the head, neck, heart or whole body can prove fatal. Shocks are more severe with alternating currents (AC), because the intensity of the current is continually changing and therefore it provides a strong intensity stimulation. It may also produce tetanic muscular contractions, which make it impossible for the victim to let go of the conductor.

CAUSES OF ELECTRIC SHOCK

Sudden increase in the current: i.e. current is switched on with controls turned up. There is insufficient time for the machine to warm-up, so the current comes on suddenly after the controls have been turned up and if the patient touches an exposed part of the circuit, an electrical shock is to be expected.

Lack of maintenance of equipment: This can lead to: frayed leads, unsound plugs, incorrect fuse use, connections not being checked, controls not set to 0, inadequate warm-up time or the current intensity being increased without due care.

Precautions

The patient must not be allowed to touch the apparatus.

All electrical equipment must be regularly serviced and maintained. This should be 4 times per year in the NHS.

EARTH SHOCK

This is caused by a connection between the live wire of the mains and the earth. An electric current occurs when there is a flow of electrons in a conductor. For a current to flow, there needs to be a potential difference, which can be viewed as the voltage drop from one region to another.

The earth circuit: the electric current is transmitted by one *live cable* and one *neutral cable*, with an *earth cable* for safety. The earth forms part of the conducting pathway and any connection (or person) between the live wire and earth completes a circuit through which a current passes. Thus, an earth shock may occur if a person makes contact with the live wire of the mains while connected to earth (e.g. resting an arm on a radiator). If a person, standing on a damp stone floor, touches the casing of an apparatus not connected to earth and with which the live wire is in contact, they will receive an earth shock.

Mains electricity is supplied by a wire at high potential, *the live wire*, and a wire at 0 potential, *the neutral wire*, connected to earth. In most cases, the current flows from the live wire through the apparatus, to the neutral wire and to earth.

This is to guard against an electric shock. If the casing was not 'earthed' and became 'live', anyone touching the casing would complete the circuit and get an earth shock.

EARTH-FREE CURRENT BY USE OF A STATIC TRANSFORMER

A static transformer reduces the danger of an earth shock by using electromagnetic induction to transfer the electrical energy into the secondary coil where earth plays no part in the circuit. The effect of the secondary coil on the magnetic field around the primary is to cause electrons to move around the secondary circuit, but not to leave it. Earth plays no part in the secondary circuit. This is an important safety factor, and all currents applied to patients are rendered earth-free by using a static transformer (*c.f.* SWD machine).

THREE-PIN PLUGS, SOCKETS AND CABLES

- The live, neutral and earth wires must always be connected correctly in a three-pin plug.
- The earth pin is the longest so that it inserts first and comes out last. This ensures that there is no time when the live is connected but the earth is interrupted.
- The wiring is identified by the colour of the insulation: *the live is brown, the neutral is blue and the earth is yellow and green.*
- The wire connected to the pin marked 'E' is for connection of the apparatus casing to earth.
- The socket into which it fits is earthed and the other end of the wire is connected to the apparatus casing. The third pin may operate a switch, which disconnects the live and neutral contact of the sockets from the source of supply when the plug is withdrawn.

FUSES

These are designed to be the weak point in a circuit. A fuse 'blows' if a current of too great an intensity is passed (see Ohm's law and Joule's law). It consists of a short wire of low melting point and if the current passing through it exceeds a certain value, the heat generated (Joule's law) melts the wire. This breaks the circuit, preventing further current flow and damage. This must be on the live wire and therefore is always broken if the fuse blows. Cartridge fuses are the most common: silver fuse wire runs between metal caps through a tube of glass. The whole tube is replaced when necessary.

For example: If the insulation on the live wire becomes worn so that the wire comes into contact with the casing of the apparatus, then the current passes by the earth wire from the casing to the earth. This is a pathway of low resistance, so the current flow is great and the fuse on the live wire should blow. This immediately stops the current flow, e.g. if the apparatus has a 12-amp fuse, using Ohm's law:

$$I \text{ (current)} = V \text{ (voltage)}/R \text{ (resistance)}$$
$$I = 12 \text{ amps}, V = 240 \text{ volts}, R = ?$$
$$R = V/I = 240/12 = 20 \text{ Ohms}$$

but, if the resistance is reduced as the current runs to earth:
$$I = V/R = 240/10 = 24 \text{ amps}$$
therefore the fuse will blow as the current is over 12 amps.

SWITCHES
The current is turned on and off by means of a switch. These mainly consist of two metal blades, which fit into metal sockets. The principle is that when the switch is on, the blades are gripped in the socket and the circuit is complete. When the circuit is broken, a spring ensures the sudden separation of the sockets and the blades. There is a switch for each light and power point.

INSULATION
The electric cable is made up of a rubber compound, which is an insulator. The live, neutral and earth wires are each covered with an insulation material to ensure that the 'bare wires' are not in contact. Electrical equipment which does not have an earth wire is usually double insulated with an insulation material; usually plastic.

OHM'S LAW AND JOULE'S LAW

OHM'S LAW
Ohm's law states that the magnitude of the electric current (I) varies directly with the electromotive force [EMF] (E) and inversely with the resistance (R):
$$I = E/R$$
where: I = current in amperes; E = EMF in volts; R = resistance in Ohms.

When a current passes through a conductor, some of its energy is converted into heat energy (Joule's law).

JOULE'S LAW
Joule's law states that the amount of heat produced in a conductor is proportional to the square of the current (I^2), the resistance (R) and the time (t) for which the current flows (I^2Rt).

APPENDIX 2

Electrotherapeutic parameters

TRANSCUTANEOUS ELECTRICAL NERVE STIMULATION (TENS) (PIN-PRICK TEST REQUIRED)

Conventional/high TENS: high frequency (150 Hz), short duration pulse width (50–80 µs) and low amplitude/intensity; ≥8 h/day.

Acupuncture-like/low TENS: low frequency (1–4 Hz), longer pulse width (200 µs) and high amplitude/intensity; 30 min.

INTERFERENTIAL THERAPY (IFT) (PIN-PRICK TEST REQUIRED)

Pain relief: 80–120 Hz, stimulation of Aβ fibres = pain gate; 15 Hz, C fibres = descending pain suppression pathways; 10–25 Hz, stimulation of Aδ and C fibres = opiate release; PAG, >50 Hz – physiological block – nociceptors.

Placebo effect: parasympathetic nerves, 10–150 Hz; sympathetic nerves, 0–5 Hz = ↑ blood flow through the area.

Motor stimulation: 0–10 Hz, smooth muscle; 10–50 Hz, skeletal muscle; 1–100 Hz, motor nerves.

Pelvic floor muscles: 1 Hz, 10–40 Hz, 40 Hz (10 min each) (see Laycock & Jerwood 1993 in Ch. 7).

Absorption of exudate: 1–10 Hz with rhythmical pumping action.

MUSCLE STIMULATION (NMES) (PIN-PRICK TEST REQUIRED)

Pulse duration, 300 µs; frequency (35 Hz), 55 Hz (pps); on/off time, 15/50 s. Treatment for 15 min × 4 daily (see Snyder-Mackler et al 1994 in Ch. 6).

SHORTWAVE DIATHERMY (SWD) (SKIN TEST REQUIRED)

Mild comfortable warmth; 10/15 min.

PULSED SHORTWAVE/PULSED ELECTROMAGNETIC ENERGY (PEME) (SKIN TEST REQUIRED)

Acute conditions, <3 W
Sub-acute conditions, 3–5 W
Chronic conditions, >5 W.

ULTRASOUND (U/S) THERAPY (SKIN TEST REQUIRED IF USING CONTINUOUS U/S)

GENERAL PRINCIPLES

Deep structure, 1 MHz
Superficial structure, 3 MHz
Acute condition, pulsed, ≤ 0.5 W/cm^2
Chronic condition, pulsed or continuous, ≤ 1 W/cm^2.

LASER THERAPY

Acute condition: pulse rate frequency (PRF), 2000 Hz; energy density, 0.2–0.8 J/cm^2.
Chronic condition: PRF, 4000 Hz; energy density, >1 J/cm^2.

APPENDIX 3

Electrotherapy: skin sensation testing

HEATING AND COOLING OF THE TISSUES

Wax	Skin sensation test – hot and cold
Hot packs	Skin sensation test – hot and cold
Ice	Skin sensation test – hot and cold
Shortwave diathermy	Skin sensation test – hot and cold

BIOSTIMULATION OF TISSUE

Pulsed electromagnetic energy (PEME)	Skin sensation test – hot and cold
Ultrasound therapy	Skin sensation test – hot and cold Only required if heating the tissues and using continuous mode

STIMULATION OF MUSCLE AND NERVE

Muscle stimulators	Skin sensation test – pin-prick test
Eutrophic	Skin sensation test – pin-prick test
Interferential therapy	Skin sensation test – pin-prick test

PAIN MODULATION

Transcutaneous electrical nerve stimulation (TENS)	Skin sensation test – pin-prick test
Interferential therapy	Skin sensation test – pin-prick test

Index

NB: Page numbers in **bold** refer to figures and tables

A

Absorption, 186
Acetaminophen, **13**
Achilles tendon, **215**
Acoustic impedance, 186
Acoustic streaming, 189
Active cancer, 216
Active tuberculosis (TB), 39, 191
Acupuncture, 78, **79**, **81–3**, 243
 -like TENS (AL-TENS), **88**, **92**, 98
 electro- (EA), **96**
 points, **91**, **96**
Ada, L., **114**
Adedoyin, R.A., **144**
Adhesive capsulitis, **197**
Ali, H.M., **168**
Allergy, cold, 63
Anaemia, sickle cell, 107
Anaesthetised skin, 80, 107
Analgesic consumption, **69**, **168**, **171**, **200**
 patient controlled, 87
Anderson, S.I., **87**
Angiogenesis, **204**
Ankles
 ankle-foot orthosis (AFO), **130**
 dorsiflexion, **48**, **63**, **169**, 177
 fractures, **144**
 laser treatment, **223**
 paraffin wax bath and, 17
 plantarflexion, **63**, **133**, **169**
 PSWD treatment, **169**, 177
 ultrasound (U/S) treatment, **204**, **207**, **209**
Anterior cruciate ligament (ACL), **125**
Anterior terminal stiffness (ATS), 71
Anteroposterior (AP) knee laxity, 71
Anticoagulant therapy, 191
Arms, upper, **153**
Arrhythmias, 80
Arterial microvascular responses, **147**
Arteriosclerosis, 58
Arthritis, 216
 acute, **48**, **180**
 Impact Measurement Scale, **118**
 Self-Help Course, **117**, **118**
 see also Osteoarthritis (OA); Rheumatoid arthritis
Arthroplasty, total knee (TKA), **69**, **87**, **114**, **120**
Arthroscopy, **69**
Ashford, R., **221**
Association of Chartered Physiotherapists in Sports Medicine (ACPSM), **63**
Avramidis, K., **114**
Ayling, J., **27**

B

Back Book, **145**
Back extension exercises, **168**

245

Back pain, 95, 121–2
  see also Low back
Baker, K.G., **195**, **206**
Baker, L.L., **131**
Banerjee, P., **115**
Barclay, V., 168
Barnsley, L., **222**
Barry, B., 62
Barthel Index, **129**
Baxter, G.D., 217, **221**
Belitsky, R.B., 62
Bell's palsy, 107
Berner, Y.N., **127**
Binder, A., **195**
Biofeedback, **119**
Biostimulation of tissue *see* Laser therapy; Pulsed shortwave diathermy (PSWD); Ultrasound (U/S) therapy
Bleakley, C., **62**
Bleeding, 7, 23, **39**, 57, 69, 191
Blood flow, 56, **147**, **149**, **151**, 189, **204**
  circulation, 216
  velocity, **117**
Blood pressure, 7, **23**, 39
Blood supply, 7, **23**, 39, **140**
Blowman, C., **116**
Bo, K., **116**–17
Bones
  growth, 164
  healing, **145**, **150**, **207**
Botulinum type A treatment (BTX), **129**–30
Bowerbank, P., **145**
Brachial plexus, 107
Brandstater, M.E., **92**
Breit, R., **87**
Bricknell, A.T., 161, **169**
Brief-intense TENS (BITENS), **89**, **98**
Brosseau, L., **11**, **27**, **88**–9, **196**
Bruce treadmill exercise test, **115**
Bruising, 70, **171**, **200**
Buljina, A.I., **27**
Burns, 38, **64**, **65**, **222**
Bursitis, subacromial, **197**
Burst TENS (BTENS), **89**, **92**, **98**
Busse, J.W., **196**
Buzzard, B.M., **63**, **169**

C

Cables, plugs, sockets and, 239–40
Calcaneal fractures, **63**, **169**
Calf muscle, **48**, **87**, **115**, **123**, **133**, 177
  ice/cold packs and, **62**, **64**, **70**
  ultrasound (U/S) treatment, 189, **198**
Callaghan, M.J., **170**
Cancer, active, 216
Cardiac disease, 56, 58, 80, 216
Cardiac pacemakers, 38, 80, 107, 140, 164
Carotid sinus, 80, 107
Carpal tunnel syndrome (CTS), **13**, 227
Carroll, D., **89**
Cavitation, 189
Central nervous tissue, 191
Cerebrovascular accident (CVA), **127**, **129**, **131**
Cervical spine
  hydrocollator pack application, **5**, **6**
  TENS application, 78–9, **79**
Chantraine, A., **128**
Chartered Society of Physiotherapy (CSP), 39, **43**, 63
Cheing, G., **90**
Chemical pain mediators, 7, 23, 39
Chesterton, L.S., **64**, **91**
Chiu, T., **91**
Chondrocyte proliferation, **173**–4, 216
Chow, R.T., **222**
Christie, A.D., **144**
Chronic heart failure (CHF), **117**
Chronic low frequency electrical stimulation (CLFES), **87**
Chronic obstructive pulmonary disease (COPD), **123**
Chronic Respiratory Disease Questionnaire (CRDQ), **123**
Circulation, 216
Circuplode attachment, 159, **163**
Claudication, intermittent, **87**
Cognitive difficulties, 217
Coherence, time and space, 214
Cold
  -induced injury, **64**–5
  -induced pain, 146

Cold (*contd*)
  allergy, 63
  therapies, 11
  urticaria, 58
Collagen, 164, **204**, 216
  extensibility, 7, **23**, **39**
Collimation, 213
Common extensor origin, 190
Compressive therapy, **225**
Continuous shortwave diathermy *see* Shortwave diathermy (SWD)
Cooling time rate, **67**
Crural ulcers, **224**
Cryocuff, 55–8, **57**, **169**
Cryoglobinaemia, 58
Cryotherapy *see* Ice/cold packs
Cuthill, G.S., **64–5**
Cuthill, J.A., **64–5**

D

de Abreu Venancio, R., **223**
de Bie, R.A., **223–4**
de Palma, F., **230**
de Quervain's tenosynovitis, **233**
Deep X-ray therapy, 7, 39, 80, 191
Dellhag, B., **28**
Deltoid muscle, **105**, **114**
Descending pain suppression pathways, 80, **97**, **140**, **150**
Diapulse unit, **168**
'Dip and wrap technique', 17–19, **20–2**
Distance from machines, 38
Dobšák, P., **117**
Doppler assessment, **117**, **149**
Dorsiflexors, ankle, **48**, **63**, **133**, **169**, **177**
Dover, G., **65**
Downing, D.S., **197**
Draper, D.O., **198**
Drop foot, spastic, **129–30**, **132**
Drowsiness, 7, **23**, **39**, 164
Dysmenorrhoea, primary, **98**
Dyspareunia, **199**
Dziedzic, K., **170–1**

E

Earth shock, 240–1
Elbow, tennis, **195**, **203**, **207**, **208**, **234**

Electrical muscle stimulation (EMS), **114**, **115**
  see also Interferential therapy (IFT); Neuromuscular electrical stimulation (NMES); Transcutaneous electrical nerve stimulation (TENS)
Electrical safety, 237–40
  earth shock, 238–9
  electric shock, 237–8
  Ohm's and Joule's laws, 240–1
  plugs, sockets and cables, 239–40
Electro-acupuncture (EA), **96**
Electrode placement
  IFT and, **139**
  NMES and, **105**, **106**, 107
  PSWD and, **163**
  TENS and, **79**, 80
Electromagnetic fields (EMFs), **50**, **181**
Electrotherapeutic parameters, 241–2
Enzyme activity, 216
Epicondylitis (tennis elbow), **195**, **203**, **207**, **208**, **234**
Epifoam, **70**
Epilepsy, 80
Epiphyseal growth plates, 191
Epiphyseal lines, 216
Eriksson, S.V., **199**
Erythema, **66**
EurolQol pre-treatment, **145**
Everett, T., **199**
Exercises
  back, **12**, **168**
  cardiopulmonary, **123**
  hand, **11**, **27**, **28–9**
  knee, **48**, **90**, **126**, **152**
  neck, **91**, **170–1**
  neurodevelopment, **100**
  pelvic floor (PFE), **116**, **119**, **147**, **154**
  shoulder, **197**
  treadmill test, **115**
Eyes, 80, 107, 191, 216

F

Faradic baths, **11**, **27**
Feet, **169**
  ankle-foot orthosis (AFO), **130**

Feet (*contd*)
  frostbite, 66
  Odstock stimulator, **132**
  paraffin wax bath and, 17
  spastic drop foot, **106**, **129–30**, **132**
Fever, 140
Fibrin deposition, 164
Fibroblast cell proliferation, **173–4**, 216
Fibromyalgia, **168**
Fingers, **100**, **168**
Finkelstein's test, **233**
Fluids
  exchange, 7, **23**, **39**, 140
  viscosity, 189
Foongchomcheay, A., **114**
Forearms, **146**, **151**
Fourie, J.A., **145**
Fractures, healing, **196**, **208**
  see also Injuries
Franek, A., **224**
French, S.D., **11**
Frostbite, **64**, **66**
Functional electrical stimulators (FES), 104
  studies on, **127–33**
Functional independence measure (FIM), **127**
Fuses, 239–40

G

Gaines, J.M., **117–18**
Gallium-aluminium-arsenide (GaAlAs), **223**, **224**, **227–9**, **233**
Gallium-arsenide (GaAs), **208**, **223**, **228**, **230**, **233–4**
Gam, A.N., **200**
Ganglion, sympathetic, 216
Gate control, pain, 80, 97, **140**, **150**
Gel packs, maternity, **70**
  see also Hydrocollator (hot) packs
General Health Questionnaire, **174**
Genuine stress incontinence (GSI), **116**, **119**, **124**, **147**, **148**
Glanz, M., **128**
Gluteal muscles, **115**
Golgi tendon, 7, **23**, **39**
Graham, C.A., **66**
Granat, M.H., **129**
Grant, A., **171**, **200**
Gray, R.J.M., **44**, **172**, **201**, **225**
Gupta, A.K., **226**

H

Haematomas, **48**, **164**, **180**, **221**
Haemorrhage, 38, 216
Haemorrhoids, **171**, **200**
Haemovac drainage, **69**
'Half value distance', 186
Hamstrings, **115**, **121**, **133**
Handmaster electrical stimulation (ES), **127**
Hands, **67**, **100**, **151**, **168**
  paraffin wax bath, 17–19, **18**, **20–1**, **21–3**
  rheumatoid arthritic (RA), **11**, **27**, **28**, **29**
Hawkes, J., **28**
Heal fractures, **63**
Healing, 7, **23**, **39**, 57
  bone, **145**, **150**, **196**, **207**
  soft tissue, **205**, **206**
  wound, **69**, **164**, **216**, **223**, **226**
Heart disease, 56, 58, 80, 216
Heart failure (CHF), chronic, **117**
Heat wrap, 6, **6**
  studies on, **11**, **13**, **14**
Heating and cooling *see* Hydrocollator (hot) packs; Ice/cold packs; Paraffin wax bath; Shortwave diathermy (SWD)
Helium-neon (HeNe), **228**, **229**
  see also Laser therapy
Hemiparetic upper limbs, **100**
Hemiplegic patients, **128**, **129**
Herrington, L., **209**
Hill, J., **173**
Hinged ankle-foot orthosis (AFO), **130**
Hips, **88**, **174**
Holmes, M.A.M., **202**
Hospital for Special Surgery (HSS), **114**
Hot packs *see* Hydrocollator (hot) packs
Houghton, P.E., **226**
Howe, T., 103, 107
Hubbard, T.J., **66**

Index

Humerus, **189**
Hurley, D.A., **145**
Hydrocollator (hot) packs, 3–15
   application, 4, **5**
   contraindications/precautions, 7
   effects/uses, 7
   equipment, 3, **3**, **4**
   heat wrap, 6, **6**
   observational checklist, **10**
   studies on, **11–14**, **48**
Hypersensitivity, skin, 58
Hypertension, **63**
Hypoaesthesia, 216

I

Ibuprofen, **13**
Ice/cold packs, 53–73
   adaptations, 55, **56**
   application, 53, **54**, **55**
   cryocuff, 55–8, **57**, 169
   effects/uses/contraindications, 56–8, **63**
   equipment, **54**
   injury, **66**
   massage, 27, 56, **71**
   observational checklist, **61**
   precautions, 58
   studies on, **11**, **14**, **62–71**, 177
IFT *see* Interferential therapy (IFT)
Immersion, ice, **56**
Implants
   metal, 38, 164, 191
   slow-release hormone capsules, 38, 164
Incontinence, 104, **150**
   genuine stress (GSI), **116**, **119**, **124**, **147**, **148**
Infections, 7, **23**, **39**, 80, 164, 191, 216
Inflammation, 57, 164, 191, **204**, 216
   acute, 7, **23**, **39**, 140, 191
Infrared radiation, 91
Injuries, 57, 164
   cold-induced, **64–5**, **66**
   fractures, **63**, **144**, **145**, **169**
   musculoskeletal, **63**, **205**
   nerve, **68**, 107
   soft tissue, **62**, **64**, **68**, 176, 216, **222**
   ultrasound (U/S) and, **195**, **202**, **205–7**
Insulation, 240
Interferential therapy (IFT), 137–56
   adaptations, 138, **139**
   application, 137–8, **139**
   currents (IFCs), **145**, **146**
   effects/contraindications, 140, **140**
   equipment, 137, **138**
   generation of, 137
   observational checklist, **143**
   parameters, 241
   studies on, **47**, **144–54**, **208**
Intermittent claudication, **87**
Irvine, J., **227**
Ischaemic conditions, 38

J

Jan, M.H., **45**
Janwantanakul, P., **67**
Jerwood, D., **147–8**
Johannsen, F., **200**
Johnson, C.A., **129–30**
Johnson, M.I., 77, 80, **92**, **146**, **153**
Joints, **46**
   effusions, 57
   pain, **63**, 177
   position sense (JPS), **65**, **71**
   range, 7, **23**, **39**
   stiffness, **12**, **13**, **28**, **29**
   tenderness, **27**, **29**, **44**, 172, **201**, **225**
Joule's law, 239, 240–1

K

Kaplan, B., **92**
Kauranen, K., **11**, **67**
Kaye, V., **92**
Khadilkar, A., **93**
Kim, C.M., **130**
Kinaesthesia sense, **100**
Kitchen, S., 3, 17, **46**, **202**, **227**
   ice/cold packs and, 53, 57–8
   PSWD and, **174**, **176**
Klaber Moffett, J.A., **174**
Kleinman, Y., **228**

Knees
  ice/cold pack treatment, 53, **54**, 55, 56, 57, 69
  IFT treatment, **139**, **144**, **152**, 153
  joint position sense (JPS), 71
  NMES treatment, **118**
  PSWD treatment, 162, **163**, 170, 174–5
  SWD treatment, 37, 45, 47, **48**, 152
  TENS treatment, 88, 90, 96, 97
  total arthroplasty (TKA), 69, 87, **114**, **120**, **126**
  total replacement (TKR), **62**, 126
  ultrasound (U/S) treatment, **196**, 203
Knight, S., **119**
Koke, A.J.A., **93–4**
Kottink, A.I.R., **131**

L

Laakso, L., **228**
Labour pain, 71, **89**, **92**, 98
Lagan, K.M., **229**
Lamb, S., **147**
Larynx, 107
Laser therapy, 213–36
  adaptations, 216
  application, 214–15, **215**
  characteristics, 213–14
  dangers/precautions, 216–17
  effects/uses/contraindications, 216
  energy/power, 214
  generation of, 213
  observational checklist, **220**
  parameters, **228**, **242**
  pulse repetition rate, 214
  radiation characteristics, **231**
  studies on, **172**, **201**, **208**, 221–34
Lateral patellar retinacular release, **124**
Laufer, Y., **175**
Laycock, J., **147–8**
Leg ulcers, **198**, 199, 221, **226**, 229
Leukocyte migration, **204**

Levine Carpal Tunnel Questionnaire, **227**
Lewek, M., **120**
Light *see* Laser therapy
Limbs, upper, **100**, **153**
Livesley, E., **121**
Low back
  hydrocollator (hot) packs and, 4, 5, 11, 12, 13, **14**
  IFT application, **139**, **145**
  TENS treatment, **93**, **98**, **99**
Low energy photon therapy (LEPT), **226**
Low intensity laser therapy (LILT), **221**, **231**
Low, J., **176**
Low level laser therapy (LLLT), **208**, 221–4, **227**, **230**, 232–4
Low-frequency electrical stimulation (LFES), **117**
Lumber spine, 5
Lundeberg, T., **203**, **229–30**

M

MacAuley, D., **68**
McGill Pain Questionnaire (MPQ), **14**, **71**, **95**, **118**, **121**, **145**
McKenzie back extension exercises, **168**
Maitland spinal mobilisations, **168**
Malignant tumours, 39
Malm, M., **229–30**
Malone, T.R., **68**
Mani, R., **147**
Manual therapy, **170**
Marks, R., **27**, **46**, **181**, **203**, **230**
Martin, D., **137**
Martin, S.S., **69**
Massage, **206**
  ice, **28**, **56**, **71**
Maternity gel packs, **70**
Maximum voluntary isometric torque (MVIT), **131**, **133**
Maxwell, L., **204**
Mayer, J.M., **12**
Medial gastrocnemius muscle, **133**
Median nerve, **153**
Medical Outcomes Study 36-Item Short-Form Health survey, **129–30**

Index

Membranes, 189, 216
Metabolic rate, 7, 23, 39, 57, 189
Metabolites, 7, 23, 39, 191
Metal, 38, 164
  implants, 38, 191
Michlovitz, S., **12–13**
Microstreaming, 189
Miller, L., **94**
Minnesota Multiphasic Personality Inventory (MMPI), **153**
Modified Ashworth Scale (MAS), **129**
Modulation TENS, **89**
Monochromaticity, 213
Moore, S.R., **95–6, 121–2**
Morphine, 87
Morsi, E., **69**
Motor points, **106, 107, 108–10**
Mouths, 80, 107
Multidimensional Task Ability Profile Questionnaire, **12**
Multiple sclerosis (MS), 121, 132, **154**
Murray, C.C., **176**
Muscles
  calf *see* Calf muscle
  contraction, **140**
  deltoid, **105, 114**
  gluteal, **115**
  hamstrings, **115, 133**
  medial gastrocnemius, **133**
  pelvic floor *see* Pelvic floor
  quadriceps *see* Quadriceps muscle
  rectus femoris, **64, 67**
  skeletal, **140**
  smooth, **140**
  spasm, 7, 23, 39, 57, **94**
  stiffness, 13, 14, **124**
  strength, **170, 232**
  supraspinatus, **114, 197, 232**
  tears, **221**
  tenderness, **44, 172, 201, 225**
  tibialis anterior, **133**
  triceps surae, **198**
  vastus lateralis, **118, 131**
  vastus medialis, **114, 117, 124, 131**
Musculoskeletal disorders, 63, 200, 206, 207, 224

N

Nadler, S.F., **13–14**
National Health Service (NHS), 47, 62, 152, 178, 231
Neck, 79, 91, 151, 170–1, 222
  see also Cervical spine
Neder, J.A., **123**
Neoplastic tissue, 107
Nerves
  central nervous tissue, 191
  fibres, **140**
  growth and repair, 164
  injuries, 68, 107
  median, **153**
  peripheral, 57, 107, 216
  peroneus, **68, 131**
  spinal, **145**
  stimulation, 7, 23, 39
    see also Neuromuscular electrical stimulation (NMES); Transcutaneous electrical nerve stimulation (TENS)
  vagus, 216
Neurodevelopment exercises, **100**
Neuromuscular electrical stimulation (NMES), 103–36
  adaptations, 104
  application, 103, **105, 106**
  equipment, 103, **104**
  functional electrical stimulators (FES), 104
  studies on, **127–33**
  motor points, 107, **108–10**
  observational checklist, 113
  parameters, 241
  precautions, 107
  studies on, **114–26**
  TENS and, **95–6**
  uses/contraindications, 104–7, **105, 106**
Neurotransmitter release, 216
Neutrophic stimulation (NTS), **116**
Newsam, C.J., **131**
Ng, M.M.L., **96**
NMES *see* Neuromuscular electrical stimulation (NMES)
Noble, J.G., **149–50**
Non-specific arthrosis, 48, 180
Northwick Park Neck Pain Questionnaire, **91–2, 170**

Numerical Rating Scale, 96
Nussbaum, E.L., 151, 231
Nutrients, 7, 23, 39, 189
Nyanzi, C.S., 204
Nykänen, M., 205

O

Obese patients, 38, 164
Obtunded reflexes, 216
Odstock foot stimulator, 132
Oedema, 7, 23, 39, 169, 171, 200
    ice/cold packs and, 57, 63, 66, 70
Ohm's law, 237, 239–40
Osteoarthritis (OA), 13, 49, 180, 181, 230
    hip, 88, 174
    knee, 118, 170, 174–5, 203
        IFT treatment, 47, 144, 152, 153
        SWD treatment, 45, 46, 48
        TENS treatment, 88, 90, 96, 98
O'Toole, G., 70
Oxygen release, 7, 23, 39

P

Pacemakers, 38, 80, 107, 140, 164, 191
Pain, 7, 23, 39, 57, 232
    back, 95, 121–2
        low, 11–14, 93, 98, 145
    chemical mediators, 7, 23, 39
    chronic, 93, 98
    cold-induced, 146
    descending suppression pathway, 80, 140, 150
    diary (NMES), 57, 117–18, 174
    gate control, 80, 97, 140, 150
    joint, 63, 88
    knee, 153, 196
    labour, 71, 89, 92, 98
    neck, 79, 91, 222
    physiological block and, 150
    postnatal perineal, 199
    postoperative, 87, 98
    Present Pain Intensity (PPI), 95, 121
    pressure threshold (PPT), 90, 153, 223
    rheumatoid arthritis (RA), 89
    self-assessed, 70
    shoulder, 205, 208
    temporomandibular pain dysfunction (TMPDS), 44, 172, 201
    undiagnosed, 80, 107
Palmer, S., 137
Paraffin wax baths, 11, 17–30
    application, 17–19, 20–1, 21–2
    contraindications/precautions, 23
    effects/uses, 23
    equipment, 17, 18
    exercise after, 23
    observational checklist, 26
    studies on, 27–9
Parasympathetic nerve, 140
Partridge, C., 46, 174, 202, 227
Patellofemoral knee pain syndrome, 196
Patient-Rated Wrist Evaluation (PRWE), 12–13
Pelvic floor, 140
    electrical stimulation, 124
    exercises (PFE), 116, 119, 147, 154
    strength, 148
PEME (Pulsed electromagnetic energy) *see* Pulsed shortwave diathermy (PSWD)
PEMF (Pulsed electromagnetic field) *see* Pulsed shortwave diathermy (PSWD)
Peres, S.E., 177
Perineal trauma, 70, 171, 199, 200
Peripheral nerves, 57, 107, 216
Peripheral resistance, 7, 23, 39
Peripheral vascular disease, 58, 63, 107
Peroneal stimulator (PS), 129
Peroneus nerve, 68, 131
Pfeifer, A.M., 123–4
Phagocytosis, 7, 23, 39, 216
Photochemistry, 231
Photon propagation, 231
Photosensitivity, 217
Physics, laser, 231
Physiological block, 150
Physiological Cost Index (PCI), 114, 129, 131, 132

Index

Physiotherapists, **49, 50, 62, 64–5, 180–1**, 222
Physiotherapy Evidence Database (PEDro), **66**
Piezoelectric transducer, 185
Pin-prick tests, 241, 243
Plantarflexors, ankle, **63, 133, 169**
Plugs and sockets, cables, 239–40
Pollicis tendon sheath, **233**
Polyarthritis, **48, 180**
Pope, G.D., **46, 152, 178, 231**
Position sense tests, **100**
Post-venous thrombosis, 39
Postnatal perineal trauma, **70, 199**
Postoperative pain, **87, 97**
Postoperative wounds, **222**
Postural stability, **209**
Powers, M.E., **65**
Pregnancy, 80, 107, 140, 164, 191, 216
    SWD treatment and, 38, 39
Present Pain Intensity (PPI), **95, 121**
Pressure pain threshold (PPT), **91, 153, 221**
Pressure sores, 179
Primary dysmenorrhoea, **97**
Prostaglandin, 216
Protein, 216
Psychological factors, adverse, 58
Pulse repetition rate (PRR), **176**
Pulsed shortwave diathermy (PSWD), 159–83
    adaptations, 162, **163**
    application, 161–2
    dosage, 159–61, **160, 161**
    effects/uses/contraindications, 164
    generation of, 159
    observational checklist, **167**
    parameters, 242
    studies on, **43–4, 46, 48, 63, 168–81, 200–1, 225**
Purdue pegboard test, **227**
Pyrexic patients, 39

Q

Quadriceps muscle
    femoris, **120, 125**
        NMES treatment, **121, 123, 125, 126, 131, 133**
            application, **106, 115, 120**

Quality of life (QOL) questionnaire, 117
Quirk, A.S., **47, 152**

R

Radiofrequency radiation, **50, 181**
Radioleucoscintigraphy techniques, **170**
Radiometry, **231**
Radiotherapy, 216
Raisler, J., **71**
Rayatt, S., **70**
Raynaud's syndrome, **63**
Rectal incontinence, 104
Rectus femoris muscle, **64, 67**
Reflexes, obtunded, 216
Reproductive organs, 191, 217
Rheumatic disorders, **207**
Rheumatoid arthritis (RA), **48, 88, 180, 222**
    hands, **11, 27, 28–9**
    shoulders, **14**
Ribonucleic acid (RNA), 216
Risk exposure, **181**
Rivermead Motor Assessment (RMA), **129**
Robertson, V., 17, **23**, 137, 164, 217
    hydrocollator (hot) packs and, 3, 7, **14**
    ice/cold packs and, 53, 57–8
    NMES and, 103, 107, **124**
    SWD and, 31, 39, **48**
    TENS and, 77, 80
    Ultrasound (U/S) and, 185, 186, 191, **205–6**
Robertson, V.J., **205–6**
Roebroeck, M.E., **206**
Roland-Morris Disability Questionnaire (RMDQ), **12, 13, 14, 145**
Rudland, J.R., **202**

S

Safety practices, **49, 180, 181**
    see also Electrical safety
Sand, P.K., **124**
Sandqvist, G., **29**
Saunders, L., **232**
Scar formation, **204**

Scatter, 186
Schindl, M., **232**
Scleroderma, 29
Scott, S., 31, 39, 164
Seaborne, D., 179
Sensation
 impaired, **23**, **39**, 58, 164, 191
 tests, **4**, 242, 243
Sepsis, acute, 191
Serotonin, 216
Shafshak, T.S., **153**
Sharma, R., **233**
Shields, N., **48–50**, **180–1**
Shingles, **222**
Shortwave diathermy (SWD), **14**, 31–51, **32**, **33**
 application, 33–5, **35**
 dangers, 38
 effects/uses/contraindications, 37–9, **38**, **39**
 generation of, 31
 hot packs vs, **14**
 observational checklist, **42**
 parameters, 242
 precautions, 38–9
 set-up variations, 35, **36**, **37**
 studies on, **43–50**, **152**, **172**, **174–8**, **180–1**, **201**, **225**
 see also Pulsed shortwave diathermy (PSWD)
Shoulders
 FES treatment, **128**
 joint position sense (JPS), **65**
 NMES treatment, **114**
 post-stroke pain, **98**
 PSWD application, **163**
 rheumatoid arthritic (RA), **14**
 SWD treatment, 33–5, **35**, **36**
 ultrasound (U/S) treatment, **197**, **205**, **207**
Shurman, J., **95–6**, **121–2**
Sickle cell anaemia, 107
Silicate gel packs *see* Hydrocollator (hot) packs
Sinus, carotid, 80, 107
Sinusitis, **48**, **180**
Skeletal muscle, **140**
Skin
 anaesthetised, 80, 107
 broken, 80, 107
 disease, 7, **23**, **39**

hypersensitivity, 58, 217
sensation tests, **4**, 161, 242, 243
temperature, **149**, **151**, **169**, **176**
 ice/cold packs and, **62**, **64**, **65**, **67**, **69**
 tumours, 7, **23**, **39**
Slow-release hormone capsules, 38, 164
Sluka, K.A., 97
Smooth muscle, **140**
Snyder-Mackler, L., **125**
Sockets and cables, plugs, 239–40
Soft tissue, **46**
 injuries, **62**, **64**, **68**, **176**, 216, **221**
 ultrasound (U/S) and, **195**, **202**, **205–7**
Sound waves *see* Ultrasound (U/S) therapy
Spastic drop foot, **129–30**
Spasticity, 57, **94**, 104
Speed, C.A., **206**
Spinal column, **151**
Spinal cord injury (SCI), **130**
Spinal nerve, **145**
Sprains
 ankle, **204**, **223**
 strains (SS) and, **13**
Standard rehabilitation (SR) programmes, **133**
Standing waves, 191
Static transformers, 238–9
Steen, M., **70**
Stephenson, R., **153**
Stevens, J.E., **126**
Stevenson, J., **66**
Stiffness, **124**, **175**
 anterior terminal (ATS), **71**
 joint, **12**, **13**, **28**, **29**
 muscle, **13**, **14**, **124**
Strains and sprains (SS), **13**
Stress incontinence (GSI), genuine, **116**, **119**, **124**, **147**, **148**
Stretching, 7, **23**, **39**, **177**
Stroke patients, **100**, **114**, **128**, **133**
Subacromial bursitis, **197**
Sugrue, M.E., **233**
Supraspinatus muscle, **114**, **197**, **232**
Surgery, 57, **87**, **97**, **222**
SWD *see* Shortwave diathermy (SWD)

Swelling, 57, **63**, **144**, 216
   PSWD and, **164**, **168**, **169**
   ultrasound (U/S) and, 189, **204**, **209**
Switches, 240
Sympathetic ganglion, 216
Synovial fluid, 7, **23**, 39
Synovitis, **45**, 164
Synthetic materials, 38, 164
Systemic sclerosis, **29**

T

Taylor, P.N., **132**
Temperature
   muscle, **198**
   skin, **149**, **151**, **169**, **176**
      ice/cold packs and, **62**, **64**, **65**, **67**, **69**
   test, **19**
Temporomandibular disorder (TMD), **223**
Temporomandibular pain dysfunction (TMPDS), **44**, **172**, **201**, **207**, **225**
Tenderness, **232**
   joint, 28, **29**, **44**, **172**, **201**, **225**
   muscle, **44**, **172**, **201**, **225**
Tendinosis, **13**
Tendon sheaths, **233**
Tendonitis, **197**, **222**, **232**
Tennis elbow, **195**, **203**, **208**, **234**
TENS *see* Transcutaneous electrical nerve stimulation (TENS)
Ter Haar, G., **207**
Tests
   Finkelstein's, **233**
   joint position sense (JPS), **65**
   pin-prick, 241, 243
   position sense, **100**
   Purdue pegboard, **227**
   range of movement (ROM), **65**
   skin, **4**, 161, 242, 243
   SWD machine, **34**, **162**
   temperature, **19**
   Timed-Up-and-Go (TUGT), **96**, **175**
   treadmill exercise, **115**
Thermal baths, **27**
Thermotherapy, **11**
Thighs, **68**, **69**, **176**

Thorax, 216
Thrombosis, 39, 140, 191
Thumbs, **68**
Tibia fractures, **145**
Tibialis anterior muscle, **133**
Timed-Up-and-Go-Test (TUGT), **96**, **175**
Tissue
   extensibility, **14**, **48**, 189
   fluid exchange, 7, **23**, 39, **140**
   injuries, 164, **176**
Total knee arthroplasty (TKA), **69**, **87**, **114**, **120**, **126**
Total knee replacement (TKR), **62**, **126**
Trachia, 107
Transcutaneous electrical nerve stimulation (TENS), 77–102
   acupuncture, 78, 79, **81–3**
   adaptation, 79
   application, 78–9, **79**
   effects/contraindications, 80
   electrode placements, 80
   equipment, 77, 77, **78**
   generation of, 77
   NMES and, **121–2**
   observational checklist, **86**
   parameters, 241
   precautions, 80
   settings, 78
   studies on, **87–100**
Trauma, acute, 7, **23**
Treadmill exercise test, **115**
Trevor, M., 103, 107
Triceps surae *see* Calf muscle
Tuberculosis (TB), 39, 191
Tumours, 39, 80, 140, 191
   skin, 7, **23**, 39

U

Uchio, Y., **71**
Ulcers, **222**
   crural, **224**
   leg, **199**, **221**, **226**, **229**
   long-term, **232**
   venous, **228**, **229**, **230**, **233**
Ultrasound (U/S) therapy, 185–211
   adaptations, 189–91, **190**
   application, 186–7

Ultrasound (U/S) therapy (*contd*)
  effects/contraindications, 189, 191, **202**
  equipment, 186, **188**
  generation of, 185–6, **187**
  observational checklist, **194**
  parameters, 242
  precautions, 191
  sound waves, 185, **187**
  studies on, **44**, **154**, 171–2, 195–209, 233–4
Urinary incontinence, 104
Urinary tract dysfunction, **154**
Urticaria, 58, **63**

V

Vaginal cones, **116**, **147**
Vagus nerve, 216
Vahtera, T., **154**
van der Wall, H., **87**
van der Windt, D.A.W.M., **207**
Vanharanta, H., **11**, 67
van Nguyen, J.P., **181**
Vascular disease, peripheral, 58, **63**, 107
Vascular insufficiency, 191
Vasoconstriction, 56
Vasodilation, **151**
Vasseljen, O., **208**, **234**
Vastus lateralis muscle, **118**, **131**
Vastus medialis muscle, **114**, **117**, **124**, **131**
Venous thrombosis, 191
Venous ulcers, **228**, **229**, **230**, **233**
  leg, **221**, **226**, **229**
Viscosity, 7, **23**, **39**, 57, 189

W

Walsh, D.M., **97**, **98**
Ward, A.R., **124**
Warden, S.J., **208**
Waters, B.L., **71**
Watson, T., **154**, 161, **169**, **208**
Wax *see* Paraffin wax bath
Weinstein, A., **197**
Williams, J., **14**
Willoughby, G.L., **144**
Wilson, H., **146**
Wilson, I., **99**
WOMAC (Western Ontario MacMaster) Osteoarthritis Index, **175**
Wound healing, **69**, 164, 216, **222**, **223**, **226**
  see also Injuries
Wrists, 12–13, 17, **36**, **234**
  ultrasound (U/S) treatment, **203**, **207**

X

X-ray therapy, deep, 7, 39, 80, 191

Y

Yan, T., **133**
Young, S., 186, 191
Yozbatiran, N., **100**

Z

Zammit, E., **209**